THE FUNCTIONAL UNITY OF THE SINGING VOICE

Second Edition

by
BARBARA M. DOSCHER

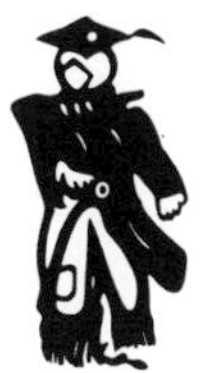

The Scarecrow Press, Inc.
Lanham, Md., & London

British Library Cataloguing-in-Publication data available

Library of Congress Cataloging-in-Publication Data

Doscher, Barbara M., 1922-
The functional unity of the singing voice / by Barbara M. Doscher. -- 2nd ed.
p. cm.
Includes bibliographical references and indexes.
ISBN 0-8108-2708-5 (acid-free paper)
1. Voice--Physiological aspects. 2. Singing--Physiological aspects. I. Title.
QP306.D67 1994
612.7'8--dc20
93-32829

Manufactured in the United States of America
Printed on acid-free paper

To

BERTON COFFIN

Dear friend, patient mentor,
and beloved teacher whose example
and encouragement have
been an abiding source
of inspiration.

TABLE OF CONTENTS

PREFACE

As indicated in the preface to the first edition, the body of factual information on which to base an understanding of how the singing voice functions grows with each passing year. The dissemination of such information is taking place in workshops and symposia, in periodicals like *The NATS Journal*, official publication of the National Association of Teachers of Singing, and *Journal of Voice*, official journal of The Voice Foundation, and in college pedagogy classes throughout the United States and Canada. Consequently, an atmosphere of inquiry, discussion, and argument has flourished, especially since the formation of NATS forty-one years ago. Not surprisingly, this exchange of ideas has produced young American and Canadian singers whose superior technical training is widely recognized.

The purpose of this book is to provide a text that describes the anatomy and physiology of the breathing and phonatory mechanisms and the acoustical laws necessary for an understanding of resonation, with the intention of establishing their functional unity. The recognition of the singing voice as a functional unit is fundamental to the development of any safe and efficient teaching method.

In general, revisions of the first edition are based on a desire for greater clarity of syntax as well as on research advancements in the field over recent years. Always to be kept in mind, of course, is that individual anatomy varies greatly, as do the teaching methods on which a "subject" in a voice science laboratory study bases his or her vocal production. As a pedagog, therefore, one must be very careful to avoid concepts that are inflexible and based on stereotypes. An educated ear is still the final judge.

The book's primary use is as a college textbook. Courses in the physiology and acoustics of the singing instrument are multiplying and may now be found even in our smaller colleges. In most instances such courses rightly precede comparative methodology, repertory for young students, and other more practical aspects of the profession. This book also is suitable for private voice teachers, for public school vocal music teachers, for directors of church choirs and community choral organizations, and for singers who want to learn about the "nuts and bolts."

The impetus for this edition, as for the first one, came from the students, who, whether in the studio or in pedagogy classes, suggested expansion and clarification of particular concepts. Once again, I would like to thank those people who provided valuable assistance with the first edition: Daniel Hoggatt for suggestions about content and syntax, Robert J. Harrison for the calligraphic inscriptions, and Patti Hay Peterson for the illustrations in the posture chapter. For this second edition, the graphics are the creation of an artist extraordinaire, David Stirts. My special thanks go to Anita Ortman for her knowledgeable advice and counsel on both content and organization, for preparing the manuscript, and for invaluable help with the bibliography.

My heartfelt love and gratitude, as always, to the late Berton Coffin. Without his patience and guidance, I would still be singing from inside a cave and practicing voodoo in my teaching.

Barbara M. Doscher
Chairwoman, Voice Faculty
College of Music
University of Colorado at Boulder
February 1993

INTERNATIONAL PHONETIC ALPHABET
(vowel symbols used in this book)

i	as in see
y	as in früh (German) or lune (French)
I	as in hit
e	as in say (but without the second or vanish vowel)
ø	as in schön (German) or feu (French)
ɛ	as in met
œ	as in können (German) or coeur (French)
u	as in too
ʊ	as in pull
o	as in rose (without the second or vanish vowel)
ɔ	as in bought
ʌ	as in sun
æ	as in hat
a	as in alma (Italian)
ɑ	as in father

Frequency key:

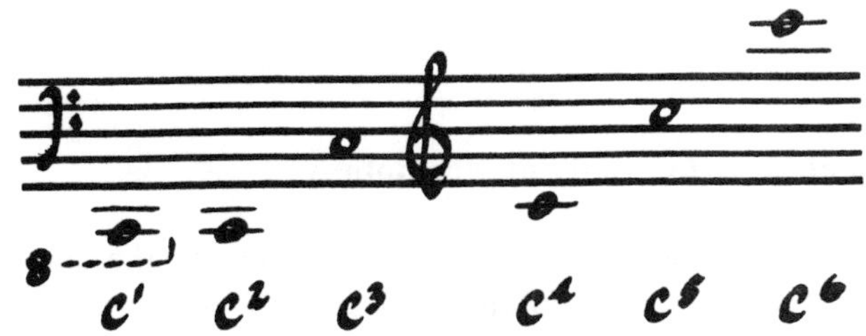

INTRODUCTION

Technique and Art

In order to produce beautiful sounds from an instrument, all musicians must learn specific coordinated physical skills. Regardless of the instrument, certain muscular actions and acoustical laws must be mastered before more subjective areas of expressivity, aesthetics, and musicality can be achieved. Emotional expressivity is difficult, if not impossible, unless what is called the "technique" of making sound is perfected enough to provide a foundation. The foundation consists of knowledge and control of the basic material of an art form, what Herbert Witherspoon, the famous American singer and singing teacher, called the "medium."

The object of art is expression.
The essence of expression is imagination.
The control of imagination is form.
The "medium" for all three is technique.[1]

The architect who knows nothing about the stress properties of the materials he uses may envision beautiful spatial forms, but his buildings will collapse because of his lack of "technical" knowledge. Form and expression are an inseparable unit, and one without the other is an exercise in futility. The musician, along with artists in other fields, must understand and cooperate with the established laws of nature. Lilli Lehmann, the legendary soprano who sang until the age of 70, believed that "a lasting art is impossible without technique."[2]

Rationale for the Study of Physiology

Music consists of notation on paper by the composer. This notation is translated into sounds by a performing musician, and the sounds produced actuate the hearing mechanism of the listener. The process sounds simple enough, but there are many unexplained or perhaps even unexplainable facets of music, both physical and psychological. Musical acoustics involve psychological as well as physical laws, since music is as much a mental phenomenon as a physical one. Acoustically speaking, progressive change is the musician's concern--the relationship between sounds.

This book does not attempt to cover any of the psychological aspects of the teaching of singing, important as they are, nor does it advocate a specific "method" of teaching singing. Rather, it is an overview of the physiology of the singing mechanism and of vocal acoustics.

> Of all musical instrument makers the voice builder is in greatest need for exhaustive and exact information about the instrument he makes, for the reason that the voice is of all musical instruments the most complicated in its method of tone production.[3]

Although the author of that statement was writing in 1935, his comments are timeless. Many teachers refuse to recognize the need to study scientific material about the vocal mechanism, possibly because of fear that their ideas will be proven "wrong," or because of feelings of inadequacy about their intellectual abilities, or even because of laziness. It is not an easy task, this study of a subject with which many of us are unfamiliar. It is so much more comforting to reassure ourselves that, after all, singing is an art and not a science. Besides, the word "science" scares most of us out of ten years' growth. There is surely no real need to learn all those difficult names like "cricoid" and "intercostal" and "formant." Singing teachers, by the very nature of this instrument, must wear many hats. Because part of another person's body is under their care, they should realize that they have a preventive medical responsibility. Would you feel at ease with a doctor who mistakes your appendix for your gall bladder? Secondly, the strenuous physical effort required of singers means that they are athletes, which makes singing teachers athletic coaches as well. And all outstanding athletic coaches have a detailed understanding and knowledge of the physiological processes of playing tennis or golf, sprinting, hurdling, or whatever. The "natural" instincts of any athlete will carry him/her only so far. If a dancer begins to have serious technical problems, an admonition to be more "artistic" is of little help.

The ideas with which voice teachers have taught singing for ten or twenty years can only benefit from a transfusion of exciting new ideas and concepts. After all, an understanding of the anatomy of the singing mechanism does not automatically mean a change in teaching methodology. It does mean that solid physiological knowledge on which to base teaching techniques will surely substantiate and broaden those techniques.

> The competent voice teacher should know the basic laws of acoustics and the principles on which the voice operates. Whether he teaches the student directly by the fact or inveigles the student to follow correct acoustical principles by parable, inference, or outright fiction, is a personal matter of teaching technique.[4]

Just as we are not happy with a mechanic who has superior hearing but knows little or nothing about an automobile engine, so we should expect a singing teacher to provide guidance based on knowledge of how the instrument works, rather than guesswork or reliance upon "instinctive artistry." In the first place, the "natural" singer who does everything right is rare and the variety of vocal problems is legion. In most cases these problems are not the ones with which teachers dealt in their own training. Methods of treating specific vocal problems vary widely. No teacher and no method has the only way to solve these problems. A knowledge of the breathing physiology, the physical action of the cords during phonation, and how the voice behaves acoustically can only give the teacher additional tools with which to work. Ignorance about how the instrument functions surely reduces the options, not only of what remedial steps can be taken, but more importantly, why they are necessary. Singing teachers are working with an irreplaceable instrument.

Once injured, no replacement parts can ever restore the original sound. Surely an elementary knowledge of the vocal instrument is mandatory.

Anatomical and Physiological Terminology

It is important to establish clear definitions, particularly of those terms which recur frequently in any discussion of physical properties of the human body. Broad terms often are used without regard for their precise meanings, and consequently there is no solid ground on which to build concepts, but merely a semantic swamp.

According to *Webster's Dictionary* (ninth edition, 1991), anatomy is the detailed examination of the structural makeup of organisms. Physiology, on the other hand, is a science dealing with the functions or processes of living organisms. At the risk of oversimplification, the former deals with the structure of the various parts of a given system and the latter with the interaction of those parts. General locational terms are:

(1) Anterior: toward the front
(2) Posterior: toward the back
(3) Transverse: horizontal
(4) Superior: upper
(5) Inferior: lower
(6) External: toward the outer surface
(7) Internal: toward the inner surface
(8) Medial: at the mid-line
(9) Process: a bony prominence or point

The densest connective tissue in the body is bone, which is held together by ligaments or tendons and moved by muscles. A ligament is a sheet of tough, fibrous tissue connecting two or more bones, bones and cartilage, or two cartilages; most of the bones in the body are positioned by ligaments. Tendons are tough tissue bundles similar to ligaments, but with less ability to stretch. They are always associated with muscles and generally attach muscles to bones.

In contrast to bone, cartilage has a firm, gristly consistency and is capable of considerable elasticity. The skeletal framework of the larynx and the trachea is comprised entirely of cartilage. The two types of cartilage used in the larynx are described in more detail in Chapter 2.

Muscle tissue is made up of three kinds of fiber.[5] Their behavioral characteristics are:

(1) Slow in response and high in fatigue resistance
(2) Fast in response and low in fatigue resistance
(3) Fast in response and high in fatigue resistance

The third type of fiber is found in the human larynx.

Apparently conditioning and proper usage of a muscle can positively affect its performance. Titze suggests that "stretching muscles regularly has been shown to maintain ample blood flow and fiber concentration."[6] Like any athlete, the singer must sing regularly to keep the muscles properly toned.

Muscle tissue constitutes about 40% of the body's weight and is used in all our voluntary actions as well as in a substantial amount of involuntary movement. In a relaxed state, a muscle is long and thin, but becomes shorter and fatter when it works or contracts. Some muscles can shorten by as much as 50% of their resting length when they contract.

Most of the body's muscles are voluntary or striated, i.e., they have a mirror image on the opposite side of the body. Each has an origin and an insertion. Origin refers to a muscle's least moveable attachment and insertion to its more moveable attachment. It follows then that the origin usually is fixed, although not always, and the direction of pull is toward it. In other words, the insertion is in the unit being acted upon. When designating a muscle, the point of origin always precedes the point of insertion, e.g., sterno-thyroid designates a muscle originating at the sternum and inserting in the thyroid cartilage. Thus the name of a muscle indicates its direction of function as well.

A striated muscle can only contract; it cannot stretch itself. It can pull, but it cannot push. No striated muscle, therefore, works alone. It is opposed in its action by one or more other muscles called its antagonist(s). An antagonist actively resists the tension of its partner or partners, the prime mover(s). At times either muscle in a functioning pair can be the antagonist of the other. On the other hand, some muscles merely hold, providing a steady base for the pulling of other muscles. This anchorage is called synergism or cooperative action.

When a muscle contracts without simultaneous activation of its antagonist(s), smooth and stable movement of that particular complex is impossible. Overemphasizing the action of one muscle at the expense of another can only bring undesirable hypertension, whereas a balancing of forces produces muscular equilibrium and smooth action. That is why finding a balanced tension within muscle groups is so vital to the consistency of laryngeal function. Examples of important muscular antagonists which behave in the above manner are:

(1) Diaphragm vs. abdominals

(2) Crico-thyroid vs. thyro-arytenoid (vocalis)

(3) Lateral crico-arytenoid vs. posterior crico-arytenoid

(4) External strap muscles (extrinsic laryngeal musculature)

The physiological behavior of these muscles is explained in succeeding chapters. "Muscles get organized to act at a given time in an orderly movement and at no other. They are like players on a stage; they have their entrances, play their parts, and make their exits."[7]

Finally, there is the muscular action called isometric contraction. In this type of action, the tension of a muscle increases or decreases without changing its basic shape (its length or thickness). Certain responses of the vocalis muscle of the vocal folds are thought to be isometric in nature. The parameters of these actions are not well understood as yet, and research is continuing.

The efficiency of a muscle is measured by its mobility, its speed of action, and its balance with other muscles, not by the mass of its strength. The ability of a muscle to react at optimum speed and efficiency declines when that muscle is overworked; it quickly loses its resilience and becomes sluggish, unresponsive, and unsteady.

The Functional Unity of Singing

The anatomical and physiological investigation of the specific areas of respiration, phonation, and resonation during the act of singing represents an artificial separation of a functional unit. A whole network of muscles and muscle-groups comprise the physiological organ of the voice. The lower parts of the respiratory system set the breath in motion, and a column of air under pressure rises from the lungs through the trachea to the vocal cords. The epiglottis is raised, the larynx is suspended in its muscular sling, and the vocal folds are stretched and brought into adduction. All these actions take place simultaneously. As the cords vibrate, the resonating cavities reinforce the sound wave in certain ways, and have an effect upon the efficiency of both the vibratory and the breathing processes.

The major parts of this functional unit are:

(1) Lungs (air or force)
(2) Larynx (vibrator)
(3) Resonance cavities (selective sound filter)
(4) Aperture (mouth or emission linkage)

As an example of the complexity of the singing act, consider the matter of vital breathing capacity. Such a basic factor naturally has an effect upon singing, but it is not necessarily a measure of the quality of tone. Additional factors of pitch, intensity, vowel, register, attack, and shape of the vocal tract also influence the amount of air consumed by a given singer, and thus minimize the importance of vital capacity in and of itself.

An investigation of the physical aspects of singing requires that these various functions be separated for didactic purposes. It is therefore desirable that a teacher of singing learn as much as possible about the muscles and their respective duties, but continue to recognize the complexity of the total act and the need for coordination of these functions.

NOTES

1. Herbert Witherspoon, *Singing* (New York: Da Capo Press, 1980; reprint of G. Schirmer edition, 1925), facing 1.

2. Lilli Lehmann, *How to Sing* (New York: Macmillan, 1902), 230.

3. John Redfield, *Music* (New York: Tudor Publishing, 1935), 278-279.

4. Robert M. Taylor, "Acoustics for the Singer," *The Emporia State Research Studies*, 6:4 (June 1958), 8.

5. Ingo R. Titze, "A Brief Introduction to Muscles," *NATS Journal*, 46:4, 16 (1990).

6. Ibid., 21.

7. John V. Basmajian, *Primary Anatomy*, 8th ed. (Baltimore: Williams & Wilkins, 1982), 117.

Chapter 1

RESPIRATION

Basic Functions

Since all living animals require oxygen, the primary function of breathing is that of ventilating the blood. This process of ventilation occurs in the lungs.

Another activity which directly links the larynx and the breathing apparatus has its origin in the early periods of human development. The larynx was at first merely a spincteric safety valve used to close the passage to the lungs, but it eventually divided, forming the vocal folds and the ventricular bands (false vocal cords). When performing strenuous activities such as heavy lifting, defecating, and giving birth, the stomach muscles, the diaphragm, and the lower back muscles automatically contract. At the same time the vocal folds, assisted by the ventricular bands, close tightly, thereby maintaining air pressure in the thorax or chest cavity. This immobilization of the thorax provides a fulcrum for the arms, as well as preventing the ascent of the diaphragm. The grunts often heard from linemen during a football game are caused by the slipping of the valve at the moment of relaxation, not during the effort itself. Such basic and vital actions naturally have not diminished, but they are examples of the use of extreme muscular tension and are not appropriate for either singing or speaking.

The last function of breathing is phonation, which includes both speaking and singing. In this book, we are concerned with singing, a strenuous physical endeavor in which the body's demands for oxygen are greatly increased. As a result, inhalation must be deeper and fuller. In addition, an adequate breath supply is needed at a specific time and for a longer duration than is necessary for speech. Indeed, both of these conditions apply to very few other athletic tasks.

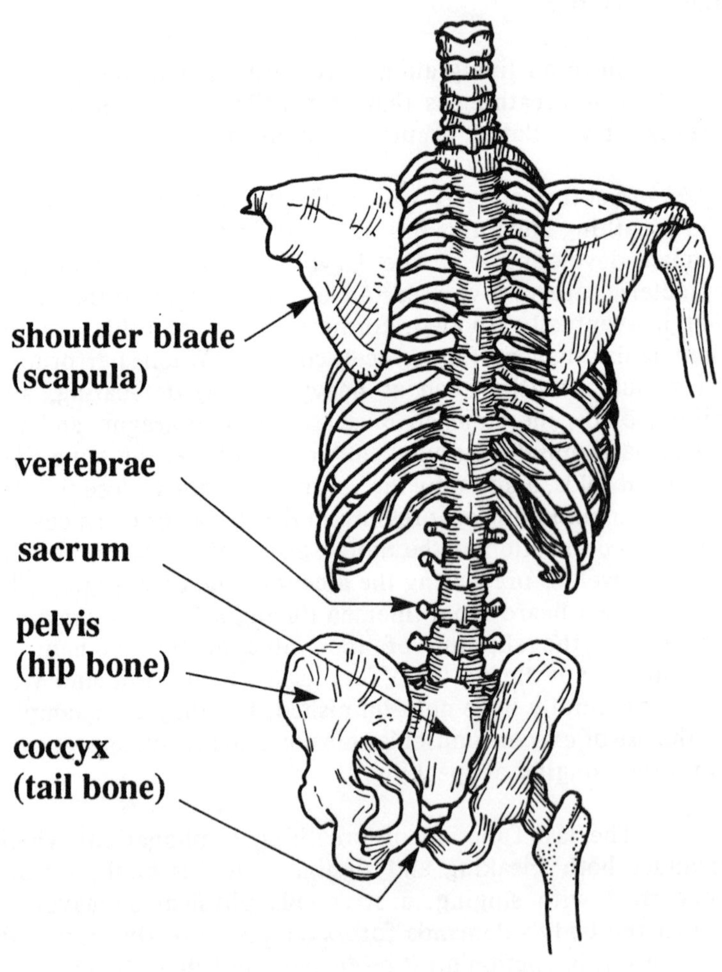

Fig. 1 Diagram of the spine and adjoining skeletal structures (posterior view)

The Skeletal Structure

The spine is composed of 24 vertebrae which are graduated in size from the smallest in the neck to the largest in the small of the back. There are seven bones in the neck (cervical), twelve bones in the area behind the chest (thoracic), and five in the lower mid-back (lumbar). Below the lumbar vertebrae is the spade-shaped sacrum, actually containing five vertebrae which are fused into a single plate. Below the sacrum is the coccyx, a fusion of three to five little tail bones. On either side of the sacrum and the coccyx are the paired hip bones which form the pelvic girdle. With the hip bones on the sides, the pubis in front, and the sacrum and coccyx behind, the entire basket-shaped structure is called the pelvis (see Fig. 1). The fact that the lower limbs are attached to the pelvis is important for an understanding of correct posture. In addition, the abdominal muscles of expiration have attachments to the top section of the pelvic girdle.

The structure of the thorax or chest is described later in this chapter.

The Respiratory System

The Lungs

Lung tissue is passive and does not exert any force other than that provided by the elasticity of the tissue itself. This elasticity is great, however, and the tissue is so thin-walled and porous that oxygen filters through it into the blood stream and is carried throughout the body.

The trachea is an elastic cartilaginous tube about five inches long and the width of a forefinger. It descends from directly below the larynx, dividing into the two bronchi which branch out into the lung tissue. Each of twenty horseshoe-shaped cartilages reinforces the elastic tissue of the trachea's walls, forming two-thirds of a ring. The back one-third of the ring is composed of muscle fibers, permitting expansion during respiration and a certain amount of stretching when one's head is tipped back.

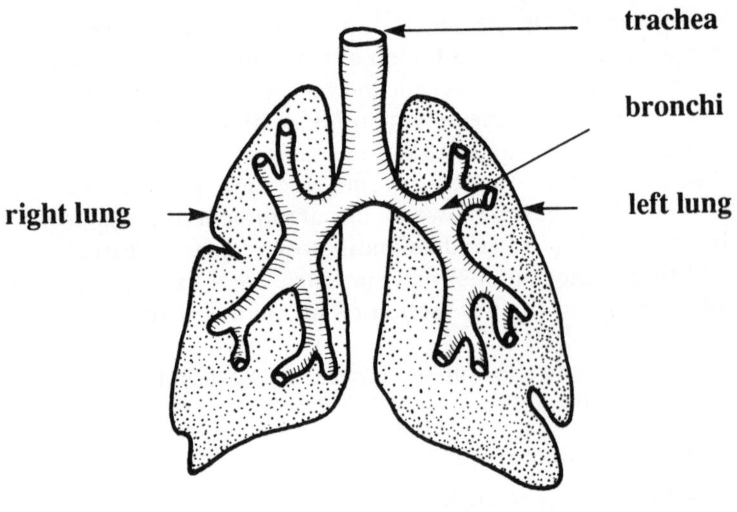

Fig. 2 Diagram of the trachea, the bronchi, and the lungs

The two bronchi divide into increasingly smaller tubes, the smallest of these opening into tiny air sacs with spongy, porous walls. Scientists estimate that there are more than 600 million such sacs in the lungs. The air sacs form clusters, the largest of which are called lobes. As shown above, two lobes make up the left lung, and three make up the right lung, giving the appearance of two irregular cone-shaped bodies.

The base of the lungs is concave and conforms to the thoracic surface of the diaphragm. The diaphragm separates the base of the right lung from the liver and the base of the left lung from the stomach and the spleen. A delicate membranous sac (the pleura) encloses the right and left sides of the lungs and makes the air pressure within the lungs particularly responsive to forces exerted by the chest cage and the diaphragm. A watery fluid produced by the pleura causes a negative pressure which bonds the lungs to the walls of the thorax.

Normal lung capacity during quiet breathing is approximately one pint, but during very deep breathing it can increase to as much as four quarts. The maximum volume of air that can be inhaled and exhaled during a single cycle of respiration is called the vital capacity. There seems to be no correlation, however, between vital capacity and tone quality, either in speech or in singing. Luchsinger maintains that two to three pints of air are sufficient to sing the longest musical phrase of 15 to 25 seconds.[1] In the final analysis the optimal use of air is determined by how efficiently the vocal folds and the resonators function with the breath stream.

The Thorax

The thorax or chest cage extends from the neck to the diaphragm and is composed of bone, cartilage, and muscle. Roughly in the shape of a truncated cone with the diaphragm at its floor, it is almost completely filled with the lungs and the heart. In the back are the twelve thoracic vertebrae, while the sternum (breast bone) and the twelve ribs on either side comprise the front and the sides of the cage. Thus the thorax has three diameters: vertical, transverse (side-to-side), and antero-posterior (front-to-back). When the ribs are lifted upward, the transverse dimension between the ribs increases. As the sternum moves forward and up, the antero-posterior dimension between the sternum and the spinal column increases. A vertical increase is brought about by the descent of the diaphragm. All diameters increase during inhalation.

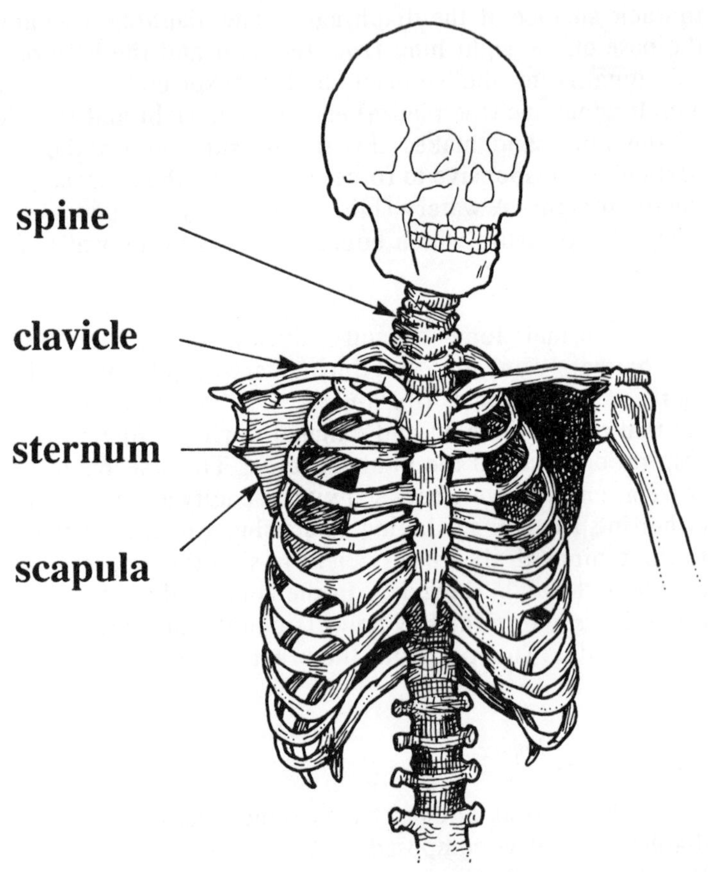

Fig. 3 Diagram of the rib cage

The sternum or breast bone attaches to and supports the clavicles (shoulder blades) at the top, attaches to the cartilages of the top seven ribs at its lateral edges, and at the bottom has a cartilaginous appendage which attaches to the abdominal musculature.

The ribs are roughly semi-circular in shape; the upper seven are almost horizontal and attach to the sternum in front and to the thoracic vertebrae in back. The eighth through the tenth ribs are sometimes called "false" ribs because their cartilages do not reach to the sternum, but merge with the rib directly above. The eleventh and twelfth ribs are "floating;" they have attachments to the spinal column, but none to the sternum. It is evident from the diagram above that the rib cage has a barrel-like appearance. From the first to the seventh ribs, the framework becomes progressively larger, then somewhat smaller from the eighth to the twelfth ribs. Because of their relationship with the sternum, however, these lower ribs have more flexibility and a much greater capacity for expansion than the upper ribs.

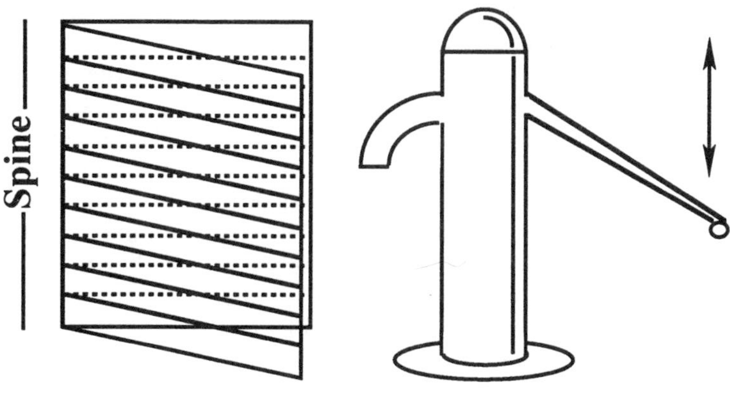

Fig. 4 Diagram of forward and upward movement of the sternum and ribs

Some authors compare the raising of the ribs to the raising of a bucket handle,[2] while others prefer an analogy to the action of a pump handle.[3] By raising the ribs, the horizontal diameter is increased. This movement, together with the forward and upward movement of the sternum, increases the size of the angle which the ribs make with the spinal column.

The Inspiratory Muscles

Inhalation can occur only when the air pressure within the lungs is less than the atmospheric pressure outside the body. To provide such a condition of lowered air pressure, the capacity of the pleural cavity must be increased, thus producing a partial vacuum and permitting the air to rush in.

The Diaphragm

The vertical space of the thorax is increased by descent of the diaphragm, the most important muscle of inspiration. This second-largest muscle in the body divides the thorax from the abdomen. It is attached to the ribs, to the sternum anteriorly, and to the spinal column posteriorly, so that its entire circumference is connected either to the thorax or the spine. Descent of the diaphragm, therefore, is of necessity initiated by the expansion of the ribs. It is a double-domed layer of muscle with the right dome slightly higher than the left and resembles an inverted bowl in shape. At its center is a large flat tendon which is thin but extremely strong. This central tendon's unusual strength is the result, at least in part, of several layers of muscle fibers that intersect at different angles. Running down from the central tendon are muscular walls which attach to the lowest ribs (costal), the breast bone (sternal), and the spine (vertebral).

The costal diaphragmatic fibers originate from the lower borders of the seventh through the twelfth ribs, interlock with the transverse abdominals (see under **Expiratory Muscles**), and then insert into the central tendon. The vertebral portion of these outer diaphragmatic fibers originates

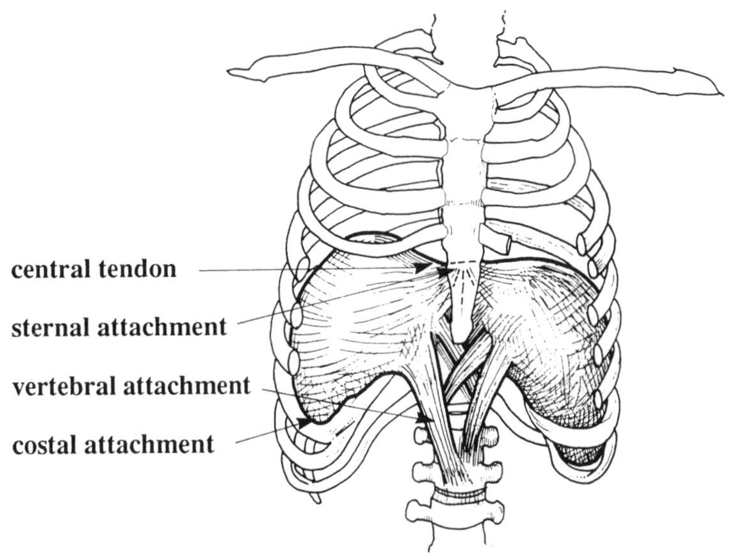

Fig. 5 Front view of the diaphragm

in the upper lumbar vertebrae (immediately below the thoracic vertebrae) by means of two heavy pillars of muscle fibers which insert into the central tendon. The sternal fibers are the shortest in the diaphragm and extend upward to insert in the front of the central tendon. Through this central tendon also pass the aorta, the artery which carries blood from the heart, the vena cava, the big vein which returns blood to the heart, and the esophagus or passage to the stomach.

When the dome of the diaphragm is relaxed, it can ascend as high as the fifth rib space, although it generally lies somewhat lower in quiet breathing. Contraction and shortening of the muscle fibers of the diaphragm pulls the central tendon down and forward, flattening it and increasing the vertical diameter of the thorax. The result is an increase in volume and a decrease in pressure within the thorax. At the same time, the descending diaphragm compresses the viscera, and there is a decrease in volume and an increase in pressure within the abdomen. A bulge in the upper abdominal wall or epigastrium is caused by the contraction of the abdominal wall musculature and is **NOT** the diaphragm itself.[4]

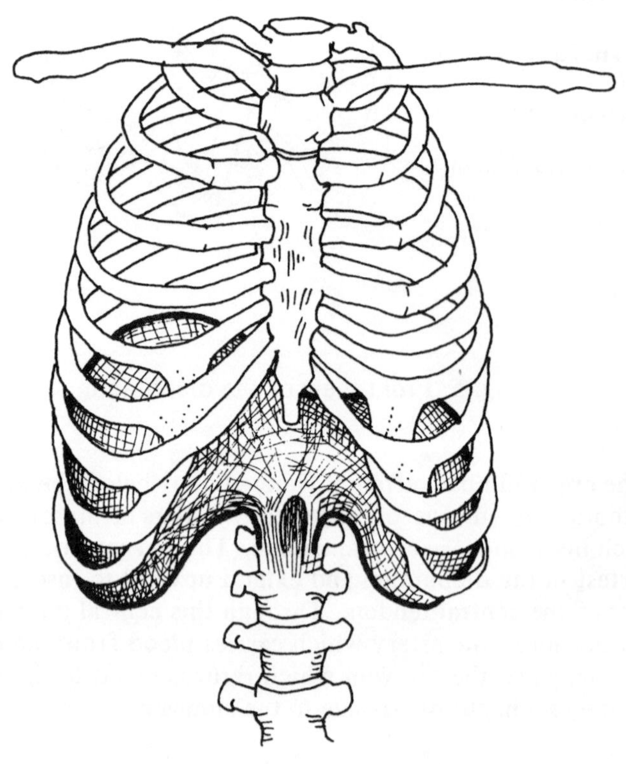

Fig. 6 Drawing of the ribcage and diaphragm at rest

The descent or contraction of the diaphragm shortens its diameter, and the greater its descent, the greater the potential force for its return to the rest position. It has been found that during quiet breathing the diaphragm descends about 1.5 centimeters, but during breathing for singing, it descends from 6 to 7 centimeters.[5] This kind of diaphragmatic action does not mean, however, that the maximum amount of air should be inhaled. A relatively small air volume is sufficient to sustain the longest musical phrase. Overcontraction of the abdominal musculature during inspiration is an excessive antagonistic action which will prevent the diaphragm from functioning properly, and should be avoided. These muscles must be trained to relax slightly so that maximum downward movement of the diaphragm can take place.[6]

The External Intercostals

The antero-posterior and the transverse diameters of the thorax are increased primarily by lifting of the thoracic cage and by raising of the ribs. There are sets of external and internal muscles lying intercostally (between the ribs). These muscles also prevent the chest wall from collapsing when pressure falls inside the thorax. Although there is still some debate about the function of these muscles and laboratory research is continuing, it seems probable from recent studies that the external intercostals are active primarily during inhalation and the internal intercostals primarily during exhalation, particularly for the kind of long, steady expiration and phonatory period required in singing.

The external intercostals have fibers which run diagonally downward away from the backbone. The contraction of these muscles pulls the ribs upward and outward, thus increasing the transverse diameter by expanding the thoracic cage sideward, and increasing the antero-posterior diameter by moving the sternum forward. This action is illustrated below.

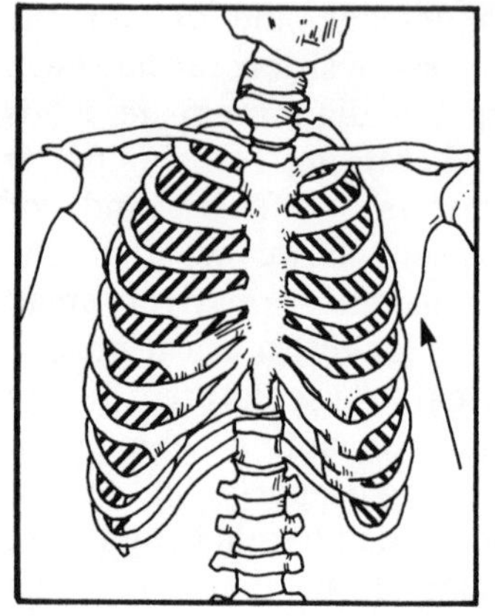

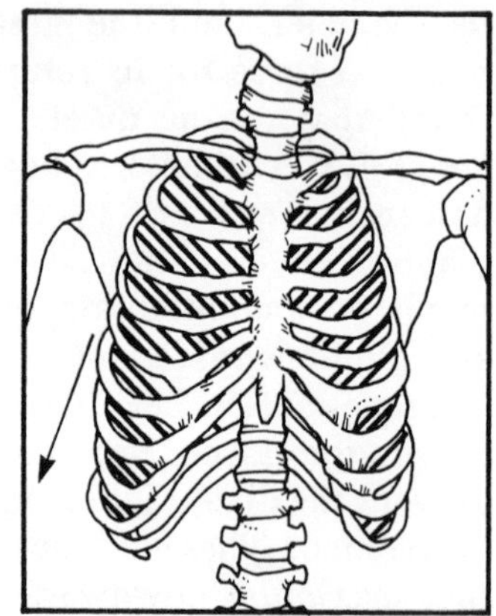

Fig. 7 Action of the Intercostal Muscles

The Expiratory Muscles

The Internal Intercostals

Antagonists to the external intercostals are the internal intercostals whose fibers run diagonally from the backbone upward and outward between each set of ribs. Their contraction pulls the ribs down to expel air from the lungs. These two sets of muscles are located at right angles to each other and are capable of a bellows action, drawing air in and expelling it. If, as many believe, breathing for singing is a cyclical process, then the inspiratory tendency must be present to some extent during expiration. Keeping the rib cage up and out as long as possible produces a flexible, balanced situation, not a tense one. A long, steady release of air also is needed for dancing and for gymnastics, but in neither case does the athlete make sounds (at least intentionally), let alone sounds which require such delicate, precise coordination of the air and the vibrator. This finely adjusted equilibrium fostered by the action of the intercostals is the work of micro-muscles, not macro-muscles.[7] The maturation process for these underdeveloped muscles can be encouraged to some extent by a regular and appropriate exercise regimen. Many singers swim or use light weights to tone the thoracic muscles.

The Abdominals

As mentioned earlier, the contraction of the diaphragm during inhalation causes it to flatten and come forward, thereby increasing the vertical capacity of the thorax. Certain abdominal organs, particularly the liver and a portion of the stomach, are displaced by the descending diaphragm. If allowed to function completely without restraints, the diaphragm relaxes and returns to its position of rest very quickly. The ribs also relax, and thoracic capacity is quickly and greatly reduced. When singing, the abdominals, the primary muscles of expiration, come into play. The diaphragm uses resistance to steady their contraction. By actively contracting when the pelvis and the thorax are in suspended positions, the abdominals maintain a firm elasticity against both the viscera and the gradual ascent of the diaphragm.

The abdominals, each a pair of muscles, are:

(1) the **rectus** abdominals which extend up and down the middle of the abdomen from the fifth, sixth, and seventh ribs to the pubic bone. The fibers run vertically |||| .

(2) the **external oblique** abdominals which originate from ribs seven through twelve, run along the sides of the belly downward and forward ////, and insert in the pelvis and the sides of the abdominal sheath.

(3) the **internal oblique** abdominals which run opposite to the external obliques. They arise from the pelvis, course upward and forward \\\\, and insert in ribs eight through twelve. They are the thickest muscles of the four sets.

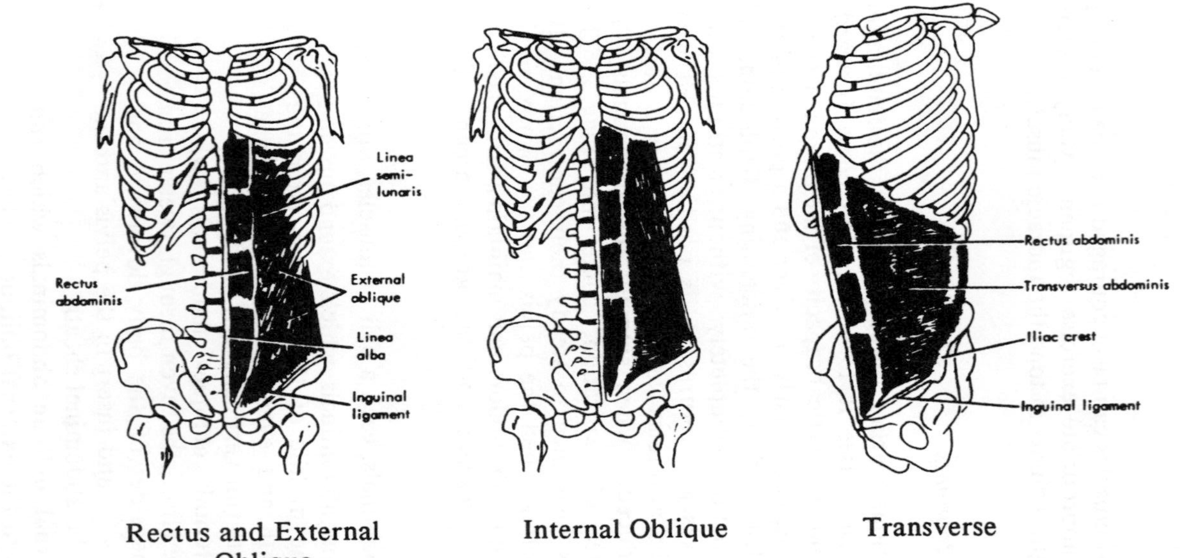

Fig. 8 Diagrams of the abdominal muscles

From Willard R. Zemlin, *Speech and Hearing Science: Anatomy & Physiology*, 3rd ed., 1988, pp. 71–73. Reprinted by permission of Prentice-Hall, Inc., Englewood Cliffs, New Jersey.

(4) the **transverse** abdominals, whose fibers are horizontal ≡. They originate from the front of the pelvis and from the inner surface of ribs six through twelve, and insert in the deepest layer of the abdominal sheath; they are the thinnest of these four sets of muscles. The fibers coming from the ribs interlock with the costal fibers of the diaphragm.

These abdominal muscles are layered exteriorly to interiorly in the order given. Studies have shown that the rectus abdominals play very little part in respiration, but are mainly flexors of the lumbar spine.[8] The other three paired abdominals help rotate the trunk, but also are the most powerful muscles of expiration. The strongest seem to be the external obliques, the fibers of which run opposite to the internal obliques.

The large abdominal muscles which hold the viscera push against the lowered diaphragm so that those lower organs may resume their accustomed places. This contraction is an active factor under the singer's voluntary control. The action of many of the expiratory muscles, however, is instinctive. Such passive factors as the gravitational weight of the bony cage of the thorax, the release of the costal cartilages, and the elastic recoil of the lung tissue are examples. In normal breathing, exhalation is an almost completely passive act as the muscles relax and regain their normal elasticity, but air pressure under these conditions is not strong enough to set the vocal bands in vibration. Certain muscles must function more actively.

One thing has become clear already: within the breathing mechanism alone, interdependence and equilibrium among the muscle groups is a physiological necessity. The diaphragm and the abdominals are natural antagonists, as are the external and internal intercostals. Some of the fibers of the transverse abdominals (expiratory muscles) interlock with the costal fibers of the diaphragm (an inspiratory muscle). This muscular gestalt or unit underlines the importance of the functional unity of this "motor" of the singing voice.

Auxiliary Respiratory Muscles

Less important muscles which may be involved in breathing by way of alignment or posture are:

(1) Pectoralis major
(2) Pectoralis minor
(3) Serratus anterior and posterior
(4) Trapezius
(5) Latissimus dorsi
(6) Transverse thoracis

Pectoralis major is a fan-shaped muscle arising from the entire length of the sternum and inserting in the humerus, the long bone of the upper arm. Its primary function is to aid in rotation of the arm. With the pectoral chest muscles in a fixed position, however, it is possible that contraction of pectoralis major helps raise the ribs and the sternum.

Pectoralis minor, which lies just beneath pectoralis major, is also fan shaped. It originates from the front ends of ribs two through four and inserts in the scapula or shoulder bone. It behaves as an extender when one reaches for something. Again, with pectoral muscles fixed, it may help in expansion of the upper chest by lifting ribs two through four.

The serratus (saw-like) anterior muscles are used to manipulate the scapula, while the serratus posterior muscles run from the ribs to the spinal column. Both sets are primarily postural in function, and any role they may have in raising or lowering the ribs is a minor one.

The trapezius muscle is shaped like a diamond with the spine as its vertical axis. Its upper attachment is to the base of the skull, while the sides connect either directly or indirectly to all the thoracic vertebrae. The far right and left corners of the muscle are attached to the ends of the clavicles. Trapezius draws the shoulder blades together, turns the head, and tilts it backward. Its primary use in singing is to facilitate correct head and neck position.

Another back muscle which receives a lot of attention in some pedagogical schools is latissimus dorsi. It is a large muscle which covers the lower half of the back, and its primary function is to extend and rotate the arm. It lies below a layer formed by the trapezius muscle, and it originates from thoracic vertebrae seven through twelve, the lumbar vertebrae and the sacrum, and the outer surface of the tenth, eleventh, and twelfth ribs. It inserts in the shoulder joint by means of a heavy rope-like tendon. Because of its rib attachments, those who believe it is an auxiliary muscle of inspiration maintain that the lower three ribs are raised. Some authorities, on the other hand, call it expiratory in function. Others, not to be left out, think it performs both ways.

The most frequently mentioned auxiliary muscle of expiration is called transversus thoracis. A thin, fan-shaped muscle, it originates from the back surface of the sternum and of ribs five through seven. It runs upward and outward to insert in the lower borders of ribs two through six. Apparently the muscle varies widely in its attachments, but its lower fibers form a continuous line with those of the transverse abdominals.

It appears likely that most of these auxiliary muscles are predominantly postural in nature and have little effect on breathing for singing. They are described here because these long anatomical words, when used indiscriminately, can be intimidating. It is a form of intellectual self-protection to know what they mean and to understand their anatomical features. Forewarned is forearmed.

The Breathing Cycle

Of the three main methods of breathing, upper chest, rib and diaphragmatic, it is generally conceded that the best method for singing is a combination of the latter two.

Upper chest or clavicular breathing is one of the few subjects on which there is universal agreement among voice teachers. It is often referred to as "the breath of exhaustion." Air is taken very quickly into only the upper portion of the lungs. The singer has little or no control over air emission, and the resultant tension in the upper chest and neck produces poor phonation and resonation. Sometimes even permanent damage of the vocal folds occurs.

We already have seen that anatomically the thorax and the abdomen are not completely separate entities. The diaphragm is attached at its circumference to the ribs, the spinal column, and the sternum. The abdominal muscle sheets are attached to the ribs. These relationships point to functional interaction. As the diaphragm contracts and moves down and forward, thoracic pressure is reduced and air rushes in. The rib cage expands upward and outward, and the upper abdomen protrudes as the abdominal viscera are shifted. The abdominal muscles relax slightly to allow for this displacement. Upon the beginning of expiration, the abdominals act antagonistically with the diaphragm as it returns to a rest position. The precise pattern of activity varies for each singer.

Contrary to popular belief, we have little or no voluntary control over diaphragmatic action. The diaphragm has no proprioceptive (stimuli arising within an organism) nerve endings, and therefore it is impossible to experience any sensation of its position or movement. There is no physiological basis for teaching someone to speak or sing with his/her diaphragm. If breathing habits need to be altered, the interaction of the entire breathing complex must be considered. Luchsinger states that " ... lateral suspension of the chest contributes significantly to the efficiency of diaphragmatic descent."[9] Zemlin concurs when he says that "although these subjects were able to control rib movements during breathing, there was no evidence of voluntary control over the regular muscles of inhalation, including the diaphragm."[10]

Diaphragmatic action, therefore, is assisted by the intercostals. If the ribs collapse, they cause a corresponding collapse of the muscle attachments with the diaphragm and the abdominal muscles. On the other hand, the abdominals are instrumental in fixing the position of the rib cage. Flexible antagonism between the distended rib cage and the lowering diaphragm on the one hand and the contraction of the abdominal muscles on the other forms the basis for steady, controlled air flow. There is coordination between the primary abdominal and thoracic muscles. The resulting expanded rib cage and large chest are visual hallmarks of the trained singer.

In the untrained singer, inspiration all too often is accompanied by excessive diaphragmatic/abdominal antagonism. The resulting tone is dull and mechanical, rather than vital, and forte singing sounds like shouting or barking. In contrast, the steady, coordinated air flow of the trained singer is evidence of slow descent of the chest and recession of the abdominal wall during expiration. There is no undue tension upon the glottis and the articulatory organs. This kind of air flow is unusual for athletes undertaking a strenuous physical activity like singing. Rhythmic breathing is most frequently used, but singers inhale at irregular intervals and must continually interrupt or reset what Titze calls their "internal pacemakers."[11] These almost continual adjustments of lung volume, rib cage volume, and abdominal volume require a degree of skill unimagined by the neophyte singer and certainly taken for granted by the general public.

Earlier in this chapter we spoke of the importance of subglottic air pressure. This pressure is the result of the flow of air against the resistance of the vocal folds, and it is a major regulator of the intensity of a tone. The primary factor governing subglottic pressure is the coordination of inspiratory effort with diaphragmatic/abdominal interaction. The resulting laryngeal adjustments regulating pitch and intensity seem to vary widely among individuals and among singing methodologies. Sundberg concedes that "... different persons seem habitually to use different muscular strategies. ... It seems that different singers use highly varying subglottic pressures, and that voice category and type of voice (or singing technique) are important factors."[12] Investigation continues in an attempt to clarify these adjustments.

Recent investigations seem to indicate that an increase in intensity is coupled with an increase in subglottic pressure ***and*** an increase in air flow.[13] Laryngeal efficiency is defined as the ratio of oral acoustic power to aerodynamic subglottic power, and "singers tend to have less glottal resistance than non-singers. There is something about the mode of vibration of the vocal folds that allows more air flow to pass through the glottis (with the same pressure) when the system is healthy and well-trained."[14] The influence of resonance factors is still relatively unexplored, but alterations in harmonic structure may produce significant fluctuations in intensity.

Airflow/subglottic pressure relationships also may vary from one singer to another and even for a single singer on different performing occasions. Evidently the optimal balance between flow and pressure is an ever-changing relationship. So long as expiration is easy and steady, this relationship remains optimal. When air reserves decrease unduly, however, and extra muscular effort by the folds is needed to maintain adequate air flow, subglottic pressure rises too much. The pressure-flow balance is upset. Rubin et al. report that "acoustically, these interfering compensatory tensions were invariably accompanied by the form of vocal inefficiency noted as throatiness or constriction. The importance of this observation in vocal pedagogy cannot be overemphasized."[15]

Francesco Lamperti, the legendary 19th century singing teacher, spoke of this muscular equilibrium in his statement on the *lutte vocale* (vocal struggle).

> To sustain a given note the air should be expelled slowly; to attain this end, the respiratory muscles, by continuing their action, strive to retain the air in the lungs, and oppose their action to that of the expiratory muscles, which, at the same time, drive it out for the production of the note. There is thus established a balance of power between these two agents, which is called the *lutte vocale*, or vocal struggle. On the retention of this equilibrium depends the just emission of the voice, and by means of it alone can true expression be given to the sound produced.[16]

Bunch agrees that support " ... is done by maintaining the inspiratory position of the rib cage for as long as possible while contracting the abdominal muscles and gradually relaxing the diaphragm."[17] Emmons describes the effect of too much air pressure on the muscles of the neck and suggests a remedy. She maintains that concentration upon the thoracic musculature often "elicits a healthy response from the abdominals even without conscious invoking of their strength."[18] Maintaining a balance, an equilibrium, is the goal.

In a 1986 experiment that has attracted considerable attention, four highly trained male singers were tested for possible diaphragmatic activity during the expiratory/ phonatory part of the cycle. Although results were not conclusive, it appears that the diaphragm may work synergistically with the external intercostals to achieve two goals.[19]

(1) keep the rib cage expanded as long as possible
(2) achieve greater speed and precision for changes in breath pressure

Some singers use the diaphragm during expiration, while others do not. Activity, when present, generally occurs toward the end of the expiratory phase of the cycle.

Breathing for singing is a cyclical process. The inspiratory tendency must be present to some extent during expiration. As a result, breathing in and singing out should not feel like opposing actions. The Italian ***appoggio*** approach is dependent upon "singing on the gesture of inhalation," another way of expressing the cyclical idea.

How does a singer acquire mobility of action and a sense of delicate balance that is the goal of controlled or managed breathing? For each singer there are individual differences, both physiological and psychological. The cyclical concept in which some inspiratory tendency is present during exhalation seems to offer the greatest conceptual and physical flexibility in which to accommodate these individual differences. The elasticity and agility of the breathing muscles are dependent upon the framework in which the diaphragm moves and upon the respiratory scaffolding of the long inner back muscles and the lower abdominal muscles working in cooperation with the intercostals. These muscles are relatively dormant in 20th century people, who are unusually sedentary creatures. In northern European and North American cultures even such broad emotional responses as loud spontaneous laughter, sobbing, and moaning are often repressed and further enervate the large respiratory muscles. Yet they must be active if the breathing cycle is to function optimally. If one cannot breathe out strongly and thoroughly enough, one cannot breathe in properly.

The Concept of Breath Support

We hear the term "breath support" used continually by all concerned with the art of singing. Its objective is the proper coordination of expiration and phonation to provide an unwavering sound, an ample supply of breath, and relief from any unnecessary and obstructive tensions in the throat. Most authorities feel that breath support is best learned when coordinated with sung sound. Although all agree on what breath support should accomplish, the "what" seems to be much easier to talk about than the "how." Richard Luchsinger is more honest about the situation than most when he calls the subject "puzzling in many respects."[20]

The variability in breathing practices is even more candidly described by Watson and Hixon[21]:

> Overall patterns differed a great deal across subjects, revealing a variety of individual styles. ... The strategy employed by a subject and the manner in which its patterning becomes neurally ingrained may depend in part on how the subject has learned on his own to use his muscular system most efficiently. ...

The researchers went on to say that differences in breath support methods were much greater among singers than among speakers. To their chagrin, however, they found that even highly trained singers did not have "correct" concepts about the breathing process. Consequently, they felt that the six male singers used in their study would sing better if the process were explained to them. The authors strongly advised against the use of imagery, but suggested that singers be told that exhalation is under a constant muscular control "that drives air from the respiratory apparatus."[22] No matter how accurate that statement, the image of "driving" air is a semantic disaster, and many singing teachers would feel that it does not promote the kind of breath energy found in a freely functioning system.

The current physical hypothesis is similar to the intuitive descriptions of the early singing teachers. If the antagonistic balance of inspiratory and expiratory musculature is working, there is a close simultaneous relationship between the oscillating subglottic air pressure and vocal cord vibration. Such a relationship partially explains the phenomenon of a full sound with no wasted air.

> The typical large chest of the professional singer reflects his learned habit of keeping the upper chest in inspiratory position, and leaving the chief work of respiratory movements to the powerful lower thoracic and abdominal muscles. ...[23]

"Support," although a commonly used term for controlled expiration during singing, is also a semantic problem for many singers. In "Semantics of the Voice," published in the *Journal of Speech and Hearing Disorders*, the distinguished laryngologist Dr. Friedrich S. Brodnitz speaks with humor and deep understanding about the importance of choosing one's words carefully. This informal lecture on semantics, the study of the meaning of words, speaks to an often-overlooked area of vocal pedagogy.

> The term "support" suggests that the voice is a kind of physical object which has to be lifted from below by a supporting force.[24]

He goes on to say that constant use of this term brings about abdominal muscular rigidity, one of the causes of many hyper-functional voice disorders.[25] One can say that the diaphragm helps to regulate and control the flow of air, but it does ***not*** support the tone. An astounding amount of tension can be generated by asking it to do so. In an attempt to induce a steady air stream without excessive tension, many teachers successfully use such imagery as feeling a cushion of air around the waist (patently physically impossible), of feeling the buoyancy of treading water, or of balancing lightly on a trampoline. The object is to keep the ribs up and out so that the abdominal muscles can maintain their leverage for steady and controlled expiration. What about substituting the term "breath energy" for "breath support?" Any practical methodology which uses the concept of freedom combined with balanced control is desirable, regardless of what terminology is used.

Since the flow of air is closely linked with the proper functioning of the larynx, it is important to note that a low, steady flow is preferable to a high, fluctuating one. Particularly for young singers, there is great danger in the use of high breath pressure before the pharyngeal muscles and the strap muscles of the neck are sufficiently developed. If the abdominal area is too stiff and rigid, the result may well be the immobilization of a region that needs to be flexible and active. Such a condition is not support, but excessive breath pressure. Rigidity is the enemy of breathing, and indeed of any muscular endeavor. Unfortunately, all too often attempts to produce vocal power originate with rigid breathing habits. In like manner, if singers struggle to conserve air by holding it in, they will not only induce an amazing amount of muscular tension, but actually will lose more air than if the attempt had never been made. Holding back air is rather like trying to drive a car with the emergency brake on.

At the same time, it is futile to try to cram as much air as possible into the lungs. Overcrowding creates adverse tension in the throat muscles and encourages a fluctuating air stream. Equally harmful is the habit of completely exhausting the supply of air before starting another inspiration. Breathe whenever convenient, regardless of whether a new air supply is needed immediately or not. Continued phonation with the last part of the available air has a cumulative and debilitating effect. It eventually leads to vocal exhaustion.

> It has become the habit of considering the breath as the only cause for a bad or a good tone. This is the cause of the eternal breath pressure with which so many singers produce their tones and ruin their voices.[26]

Considering the variability of breathing practices, it is probably well-advised to admit that from an empirical point of view, and probably from a scientific one as well, there is no set formula for ideal breathing that will fit every singer. "The singing teacher who tries to impose on all pupils *one* form of breathing will only risk the ruin of promising voices."[27] When a voice teacher has a good basic understanding of the physiology of the breathing apparatus, there is a realization that there are several ways to accomplish one's goal. If the antagonistic balancing of inspiratory and expiratory musculature can be achieved, a free, steady stream of air is the beneficial result.

NOTES

1. Richard Luchsinger and Godfrey E. Arnold, *Voice-Speech-Language* (Belmont, Ca.: Wadsworth Publishing, 1965), 19.

2. Basmajian, op. cit., 48.

3. Meribeth Bunch, *Dynamics of the Singing Voice* (New York: Springer-Verlag, 1982), 29.

4. Johan Sundberg and Rolf Leanderson, "Phonatory Breathing--Physiology Behind Voice Pedagogy: A Tutorial," *Journal of Research in Singing*, 10:1 (1986), 3-21.

5. Cited in D. Ralph Appelman, *The Science of Vocal Pedagogy* (Bloomington, IN: Indiana University Press, 1967), 33 (from O.L. Wade, "Movements of the Thoracic Cage and Diaphragm in Respiration," *Journal of Physiology*, Vol. 124, 1954; 193-212).

6. Bunch, op. cit., 47.

7. Macro is defined by *Webster's Dictionary* as excessively developed, in this case a muscle that has been used extensively from an early age. Examples

are the diaphragm or the chewing muscles. Micro literally means small, but in this case, we use it to mean needing development. In our couch-potato society, the intercostals and such neck muscles as the trapezius are examples of micro-muscles.

8. Bunch, op. cit., 37.

9. Luchsinger and Arnold, op. cit., 5.

10. Willard R. Zemlin, *Speech and Hearing Science*, Third Edition (Englewood Cliffs, NJ: Prentice-Hall, 1988), 62.

11. Ingo Titze, "Some Notes on Breath Control in Singing," *NATS Journal*, 43:2 (1986), 28.

12. Johan Sundberg, *The Science of the Singing Voice* (DeKalb, IL: Northern Illinois University Press, 1987), 25, 36.

13. H. K. Schutte, "Efficiency of Professional Singing Voices in Terms of Energy Ratio," *Folia Phoniatrica*, 36:6 (1984), 268. See also Ingo Titze, "Glottal Resistance," *NATS Journal*, 48:4 (1992), 51.

14. Ingo Titze, "Glottal Resistance," *NATS Journal*, 48:4 (1992), 51.

15. H. J. Rubin, M. Le Cover, W. Vennard, "Vocal Intensity, Subglottic Pressure and Air Flow Relationships in Singers," *Folia Phoniatrica*, 19:6 (1967), 397.

16. Francesco Lamperti, *The Art of Singing* (New York: G. Schirmer, ca. 1890), 25.

17. Bunch, op. cit., 47.

18. Shirlee Emmons, "Breathing for Singing," *Journal of Voice*, 2:1 (1988), 31.

19. Rolf Leanderson, Johan Sundberg, and Curt von Euler, "Role of Diaphragmatic Activity During Singing: A Study of Transdiaphragmatic Pressures," *Journal of Applied Physiology*, 62:1 (1987), 264.

20. Luchsinger and Arnold, op. cit., 13.

21. Peter J. Watson and Thomas J. Hixon, "Respiratory Kinematics in Classical (Opera) Singing," *Journal of Speech and Hearing Research*, 28:1 (1985), 115-116.

22. Ibid., 122.

23. Luchsinger and Arnold, op. cit., 14.

24. Friedrich S. Brodnitz, "Semantics of the Voice," *Journal of Speech and Hearing Disorders*, 32:4 (1967), 325-330.

> Dr. Brodnitz mentions two other directives that are too frequently used by unmindful voice teachers. "Speak from the diaphragm" is a physiologically unsound concept, as we have seen. "Project the voice," he says, sounds as if one is throwing a stone or a javelin as far as possible by the use of great force. "The carrying power of a voice is the result of the coordination of breath control, vocal fold adjustment, and 'free resonance'."

25. Ibid., 327-328.

26. Lehmann, op. cit., 224.

27. Friedrich S. Brodnitz, *Keep Your Voice Healthy*, Second Edition (Boston: College-Hill Press, 1988), 137.

Chapter 2

ANATOMY OF THE LARYNX

At the risk of oversimplification, it can be said that the 18th century was the century of breathing, the 19th that of resonance, and the 20th that of the larynx. It is certainly true that purely scientific investigation into the physical characteristics of the larynx and the manner in which phonation takes place has been pursued primarily in this century and has shed much light upon how the singing instrument works. Because of the complexity of the larynx and particularly of its functional unity with the breathing mechanism and the resonating cavities, there remain many areas of uncertainty. Research continues to be done.

The larynx is positioned in the throat by a series of suspensory muscles. It is anchored from below by muscular attachments to the sternum and the clavicles. Its lowest cartilage, the cricoid, is also stabilized by a ligamental attachment to the first ring of the trachea. At the top it is suspended from the hyoid bone.

The Hyoid Bone and Major Cartilages of the Larynx

The Hyoid Bone

The hyoid bone is horseshoe-shaped with the opening at the back. Since it is not attached to any other bone in the skeleton, but is kept in position by a complex system of muscles and ligaments, it is extremely mobile. Muscles of the tongue and chin attach to the hyoid from above and front, while muscles from the temporal bone and the styloid processes (both located behind the ear) attach from above and behind. Muscles running from the larynx to the sternum, clavicles, and the scapula attach from below. All of these muscles, sometimes called "strap muscles" of the neck, are discussed in more detail later in this chapter.

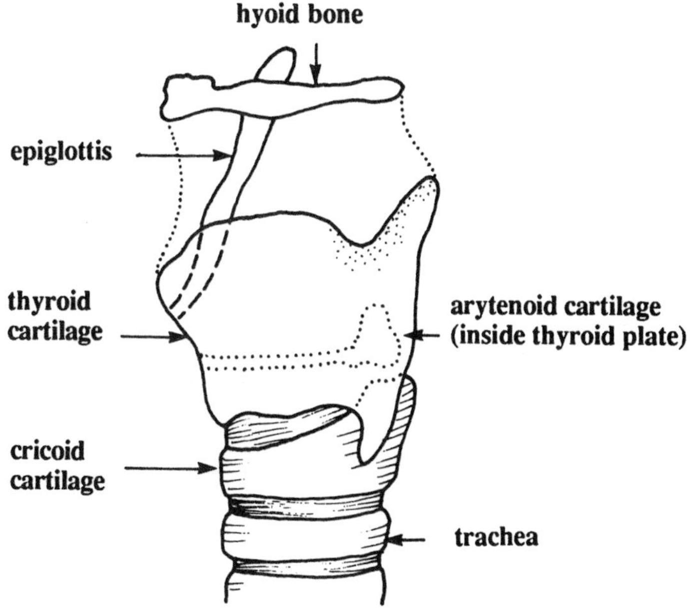

Fig. 9 Schematic Sideview of the Larynx

Cartilages of the Larynx

The larynx, consisting of a series of cartilages, is essentially a valve between the trachea and the root of the tongue. This valve can be used to make sounds, but it also can be closed off entirely when the epiglottis, like the lid of a box, lowers to protect the trachea or windpipe during swallowing. The old saying about "swallowing down the wrong pipe" is a literal one. Food or liquid intended for the esophagus, the tube leading to the stomach, finds its way past the epiglottis and into the trachea. The resultant coughing is an attempt to expel that foreign material.

There are four major cartilages of the larynx: the cricoid, the thyroid, the two arytenoids, and the epiglottis; and two adjunct cartilages: the corniculates and the cuneiforms. Beginning at the bottom, the cricoid cartilage sits on top of and is attached to the uppermost ring of the trachea. It is round and shaped like a signet ring, broad in back and narrow in front. In size it is just big enough to admit a forefinger (not that such an action is advised).

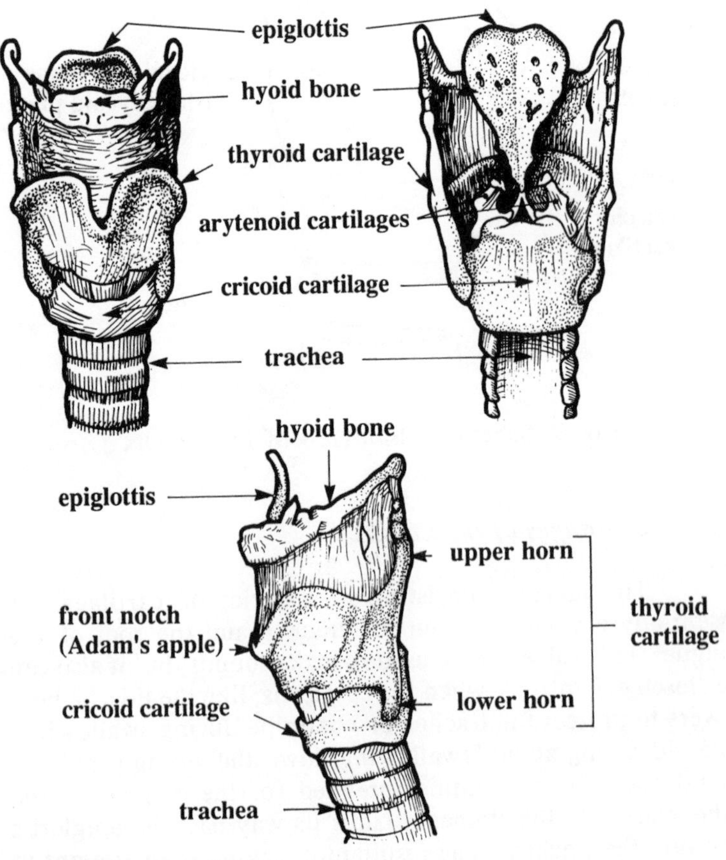

Fig. 10 Cartilages of the Larynx

The thyroid cartilage is composed of two plates which fuse together in front at an acute angle and flair apart posteriorly to form a **V**. Its shape is like that of a shield. The apex of this cartilage is commonly called the Adam's apple. The lower horns of the thyroid are joined to the back lower part of the cricoid in such a way as to allow a rocking action as well as a front-to-back sliding motion by either or both cartilages. The upper horns of the thyroid cartilage are loosely jointed to the tips of the hyoid bone (See Fig. 10).

Mounted upon the upper edge of the back of the cricoid cartilage and shaped like triangular pyramids are the two arytenoid cartilages. The crico-arytenoid joints are capable of extremely complex movements. They can glide in medial and lateral directions, rotate, and slide forward and backward. Any combination of these movements can occur simultaneously! Each arytenoid cartilage has three processes or tips, the vocal process which projects forward, the muscular process which projects down and back, and the corniculate cartilage which forms the apex or top of the structure. Attached to the vocal processes are the vocal folds, and attached to the muscular processes are those muscles which open and close the folds (See Fig. 11).

Of the two adjunct cartilages, the paired corniculate cartilages are vestigial structures and no longer have a function. The cuneiform cartilages are paired wedge-shaped rods of elastic material and are imbedded in the ary-epiglottic folds. They help form the entrance to the larynx, a function discussed in more detail under **The Resonance Cavities** in Chapter 6.

The cricoid and thyroid cartilages are composed of hyaline, a bluish-white, rather translucent substance of great firmness and strength as well as elasticity. With advancing age, it sometimes loses its color and turns yellow and cloudy. Calcification or even ossification (becoming bone) may occur. Although there is conjecture that poor nutrition causes such a change, there is as yet no solid proof to support that theory.

The main part of the arytenoid cartilage consists of hyaline material, but its three processes are made of much more elastic material.

The epiglottis, composed entirely of this same extremely elastic yellow cartilaginous material, is in the shape of a leaf whose stem is attached to the inner surface of the front of the thyroid cartilage just above the insertion of the vocal folds (See Fig. 10). During swallowing, it is partially pulled down by the aryepiglottic folds[1] and partially pushed down by the back of the tongue. Although the general shape of the epiglottis is that of a leaf, each one differs slightly in size and contour. The fibrous consistency of this cartilage makes it similar to the ear and parts of the nose, which also vary from one individual to the next. Even those cartilages made of hyaline material may vary somewhat in shape. "One outstanding structural feature of the larynx is asymmetry. This is especially true of the thyroid cartilage."[2] Another noted voice scientist believes that larynxes, like faces, are seldom perfectly symmetrical.[3]

Throat specialists ask their patients to say /**i**/, not /**a**/, because the tongue and with it the epiglottis is farther forward on /**i**/, permitting them a clearer view of the larynx. What are the implications for changes in the resonating area immediately above the larynx, that small resonator formed by the aryepiglottic folds? Zemlin maintains that the position of the epiglottis "may modify the laryngeal tone by producing changes in the size and shape of the laryngeal cavity."[4] Appelman says that the position of the epiglottis is controlled primarily by movements of the tongue root and that variations of position cause changes in the dimensions of the laryngeal vestibule during the phonation of each vowel.[5] The undesirability of excessive tension in such "false" elevators as the tongue root is examined later in this chapter when the extrinsic muscles of the larynx and optimum laryngeal positioning are reviewed.

Definition of Intrinsic and Extrinsic Muscles

Before we discuss the muscles of the larynx, it is important to differentiate between intrinsic and extrinsic. The intrinsic muscles of the larynx move its parts with relation to each other and have both attachments within the larynx, whereas the extrinsic muscles have at least one attachment to structures outside the larynx and generally move the larynx as a whole. All of these muscles are paired.

The Intrinsic Muscles

The Vocal Folds

Probably the most talked about but least understood organs of the larynx are the vocal folds. They consist of two wedge-shaped bundles of muscles with ligamental edges, the whole covered by a mucous membrane. These folds originate on the inner surface of the thyroid notch and attach to the arytenoid cartilages posteriorly. Their anatomical name is the thyro-arytenoids, **thyro** for the place of origin and **arytenoid** for the place of insertion. The vocalis or internal thyro-arytenoid forms the main mass of the folds and its primary function is as an isometric tensor; it can vary frequency and manner of vibration by partial or segmental contraction. The mucous membrane which covers the folds is called the conus elasticus. It fits loosely, like the skin on the back of one's hand, so it is possible for the edges or vocal ligaments to vibrate relatively independently of the main muscle mass. Although the dimensions of the glottis (the space between the folds) are highly variable between individuals and even within a single person, the front or membranous portion of the vocal folds takes up about two-thirds of their total length. The remaining one-third is called the cartilaginous section because its border is formed by the vocal processes (tips) of the arytenoid cartilages. The shape and size of the glottis is influenced by the rotation of the arytenoid cartilages, by the sub-glottic air pressure, by the transglottal air flow, and by the contraction of the laryngeal muscles.

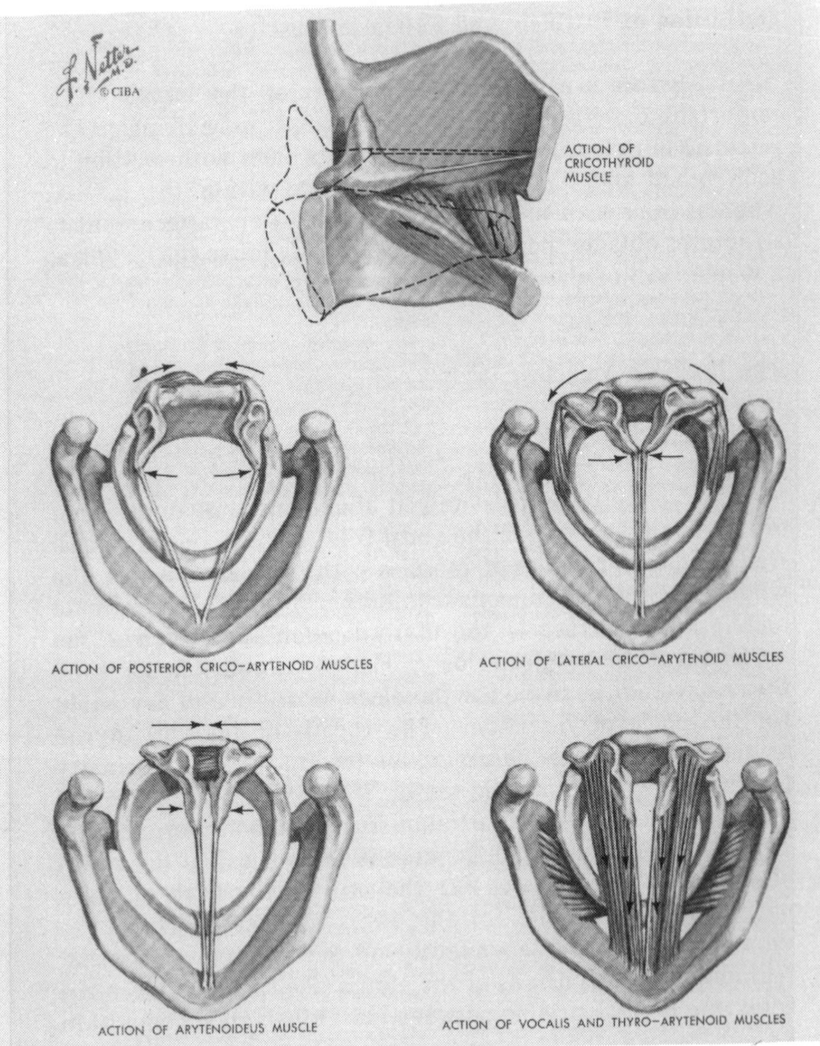

Fig. 11 Action of the Crico-Arytenoid Muscles and the Thyro-Arytenoid Vocal Folds

The folds generally are a light pink in color with white ligamental edges. In people with laryngitis, they become bright red with distended blood vessels. The morphology or physical structure of the vocal folds is examined in greater detail in the appendix when the causes of vocal nodules are investigated.

It is apparent that the vocal folds are an extremely complex tensing and relaxing mechanism. As laboratory research continues, the intricate nature of these two tiny wedges of muscle becomes even more evident. The vocal folds seem to be multi-layered muscles, and their versatility of function is astonishing. They can shorten themselves, contract laterally, vary both the length and the thickness of a vibrating segment, and even make part of themselves tense while the rest is relaxed. No man-made instrument can equal this kind of versatility.

The False Vocal Folds

Directly above the vocal folds are two narrow horizontal cavities called the ventricles of Morgagni, and above them are two fleshy folds with down-turned borders, the false vocal cords. The ventricles contain glands which secrete lubricating material for the true vocal folds to defend against excessive friction during phonation. The false folds have few muscle fibers so that tension, mass, and length are difficult to control. These folds take no part in phonation: their primary function is a valvular one, in cooperation with the true cords, to prevent the escape of air from the lungs. This kind of important biological activity was described at the beginning of Chapter 1.

The Crico-Thyroid Muscle

This muscle has its origin in the front and the side of the cricoid cartilage and its insertion in the front of the lower horn and in the lower border of the thyroid. It is a fan-shaped muscle, broader at the top than at the bottom, as shown in Figure 14.

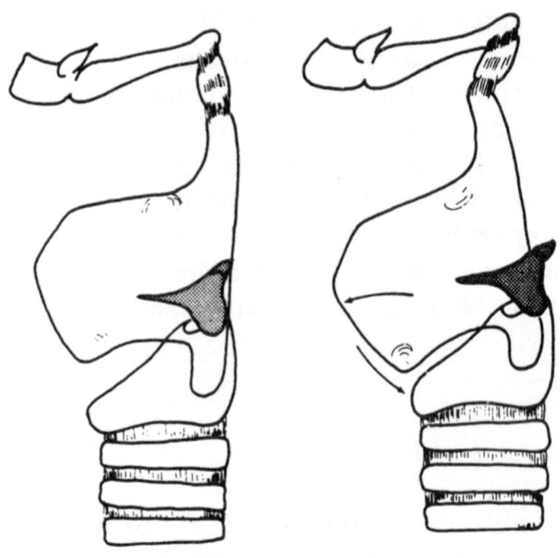

Fig. 12 Contraction of the Crico-thyroid and its Effect upon the Thyroid Cartilage (Forward tilting of the thyroid cartilage increases the front-to-back distance of the larynx, and thus places the vocal folds under increased tension)

Willard R. Zemlin, *Speech and Hearing Science: Anatomy & Physiology*, 3rd ed., 1988, p. 112. Reprinted by permission of Prentice-Hall, Inc., Englewood Cliffs, New Jersey.

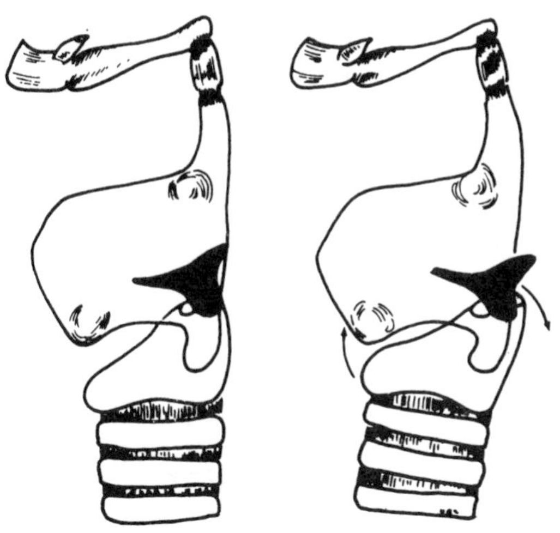

Fig. 13 Contraction of the Crico-thyroid and its effect upon the Cricoid cartilage (The cricoid cartilage rotates down in back and up in front, thereby increasing the distance between the arytenoid cartilages and the thyroid cartilage and stretching the vocal folds)

Willard R. Zemlin, *Speech and Hearing Science: Anatomy & Physiology*, 3rd ed., 1988, p. 112. Reprinted by permission of Prentice-Hall, Inc., Englewood Cliffs, New Jersey.

The primary function of the crico-thyroid is as a vocal fold stretcher. It can tilt the thyroid cartilage forward, thereby increasing the distance between the front of the vocal folds at the thyroid notch and the arytenoid cartilages posteriorly. The vocal folds are elongated and tensed.

If the thyroid cartilage is relatively fixed by the action of the extrinsic laryngeal muscles (see **Extrinsic Muscles** later in this chapter), crico-thyroid contraction will raise the front of the cricoid cartilage and lower it posteriorly. It is clear from Figs. 12 and 13 that either action will result in alterations in vocal fold tension and/or length.

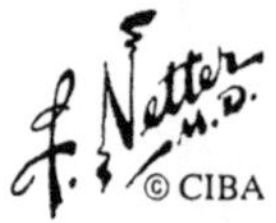

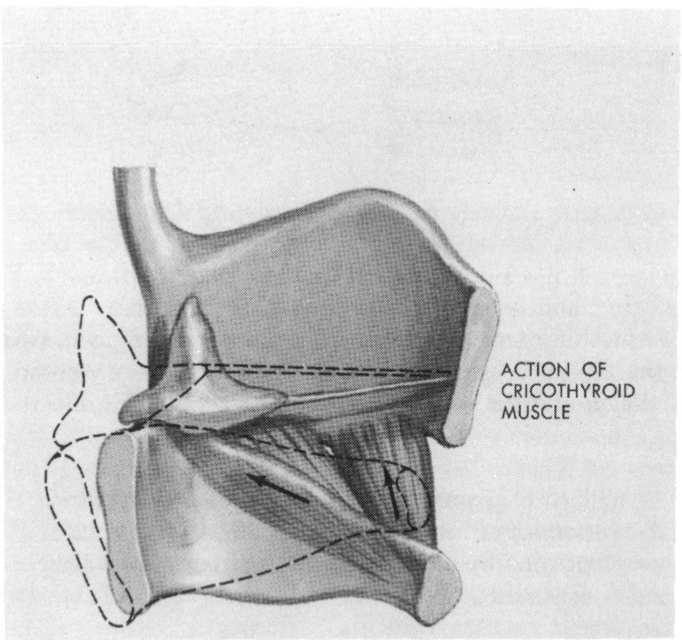

Fig. 14 Action of the Crico-thyroid Muscle

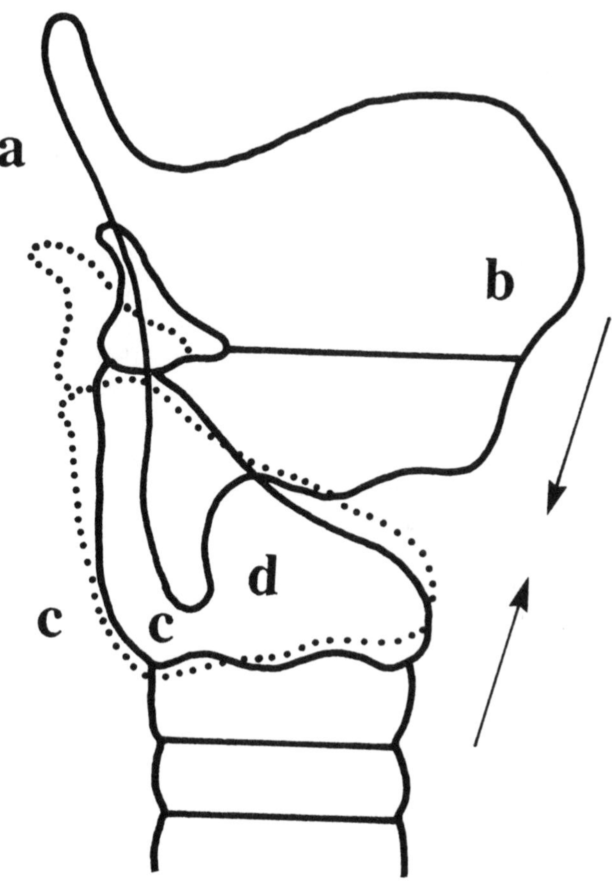

Fig. 15 Action of the Crico-thyroid Muscle
(after Garcia)

It is interesting to note that Luchsinger (1965), Saunders (1964), and Gould (1971) believe that, although the thyroid cartilage moves forward and down slightly, the major response to crico-thyroid contraction is by the cricoid cartilage, which has no muscular connections to the skeleton, as does the thyroid.[6] Manuel Garcia's 1894 book has a diagram showing the contraction of the crico-thyroid muscle and the resultant movement of the cricoid cartilage, which is a rocking motion that tilts the cartilage up in front and down in back.[7] It directly parallels that depicted by Frank Netter, M.D. Both are shown in Figs. 14 and 15.

The primary function of the crico-thyroid muscle is that of crude, external vocal fold tension by stretching. The vocalis muscle performs the more refined and precise tensing functions, but the two sets of muscles must work together. As a result of its function as a stretcher, the crico-thyroid is important in determining pitch. Sonninen (1956) showed by lateral radiography that the cords become longer with rising pitch.[8] Minoru Hirano, the leading expert on vocal fold morphology (the structure of an organism), lists the following vocal fold changes in shape as a result of the crico-thyroid/vocalis antagonism.[9]

Crico-thyroid	**Vocalis**
folds elongated	folds shortened
folds thinned	folds thickened
edges of folds sharpened	edges of folds rounded

It seems probable, then, that pitch is determined not only by total cord length, but also by the length and breadth of the segment which may be vibrating, a factor which is generally under the control of the vocalis muscle. Further research is needed.

The Crico-Arytenoid Muscles

There are three major kinds of crico-arytenoid muscles. Two are adductors and one is an abductor. To adduct means to bring together or approximate. To abduct means to pull apart or separate.

The single abductor of the vocal folds is the posterior crico-arytenoid (See upper left drawing in Fig. 11). It is a paired, broad, fan-shaped muscle which originates on the back surface of the cricoid cartilage, then narrows for insertion into the muscular process of the arytenoid cartilage. When the vocal folds are abducted, the space between them is called the glottis.

The lateral crico-arytenoid is the primary adductor and is a direct antagonist to the posterior crico-arytenoid abductor. It extends from the upper border on either side of the cricoid cartilage to the muscular process of each arytenoid cartilage. This muscle adducts the greater part of the vocal folds, leaving open a small triangular space or chink between the arytenoid cartilages (See upper right drawing in Fig. 11). The action of the lateral crico-arytenoid is termed "medial compression."

The inter-arytenoids extend from the back surface of one arytenoid cartilage to the corresponding part of the other arytenoid, forming a muscular **X** and drawing the tips of the arytenoids together to complete the closure (See lower left drawing in Fig. 11). Late development of the inter-arytenoids is common during the teen years, especially in young women, and the resultant triangular opening between the arytenoids is called "the mutational chink." Such a condition during phonation produces breathiness of tone and is particularly common in junior high and early high school voices. Vennard describes the typical sound as that of a clear little voice, accompanied by the rustling of "wild air" through the chink.[10] Maturation will cure the problem, but the cords should not be forced into a clear phonation posture before proper muscular development has taken place. The continual use of /**i**/ and /**e**/ vowels to bring the cords together more firmly may temporarily alleviate the breathiness, but is a dangerous way of correcting a natural physical condition. Constant use of /**i**/ and /**e**/ requires a higher breath pressure and greater muscular resistance in the vocal folds. Both put unnecessary and potentially harmful strain on growing young muscles. The undesirable resonance implications of using these closed front vowels too much, especially with female voices, will become apparent in the chapter on vowel formants, especially in the section on the soprano voice. The normal vocalization of the young voice, with particular attention to a steady, energized breath stream and to efficient resonation techniques, will produce healthier long-range results.

It is apparent that there are two primary pairs of intrinsic muscles in the larynx. The flexor (vocalis) works with the tensor (crico-thyroid), and the main adductor (lateral crico-arytenoid) is the antagonist of the abductor (posterior crico-arytenoid). It should be noted, however, that the lateral crico-arytenoid as the primary adductor also works synergistically with the crico-thyroid. As the crico-thyroid stretches the cords and creates greater longitudinal tension, the vocal folds tend to gap. More medial compression is needed for a firm adduction, which is the job of the lateral crico-arytenoids.

The Extrinsic Muscles

The network of muscles which provides an elastic scaffolding for the larynx is called the suspensory mechanism. Some authors call this complex the strap muscles. These extrinsic muscles are in large part responsible for the position and relative stability of the larynx. They also play an important role in controlling the length and tension of the vocal folds, especially the sterno-thyroid depressor, another antagonist of the crico-thyroid stretcher.[11]

As early as 1959, William Vennard complained about how few articles there were on the extrinsic muscles. The situation has not changed materially since then. Vennard went on to say that he had formerly believed that during artistic singing the intrinsic muscles did most of the laryngeal work, while the extrinsic musculature simply relaxed. He no longer held that view, but felt that the swallowing muscles are the only ones that must relax.[12]

Anatomically, the extrinsic muscles may be classed as supra-hyoid (above) and infra-hyoid (below), although some authors prefer to call the entire unit the hyoid-larynx complex. Although the latter is a descriptive name anatomically, the functional duties of these muscles describe them more accurately.

The four major supra-hyoid muscles are the digastric, the stylo-hyoid, the mylo-hyoid, and the genio-hyoid. Many of these muscles are what can be called "false elevators"; that is, their use produces undesirable tension in the tongue and the pharyngeal area. The digastric muscle has two sections, one running from under the chin to the hyoid and the other from the mastoid process behind the ear to the hyoid. Although the front part is a tongue muscle and the back part is a swallowing muscle, both strongly draw the hyoid bone up in preparation for deglutition. The back section, together with the stylo-hyoid, is a major factor in the final pharyngeal phase of swallowing. The stylo-hyoid originates from the styloid process and runs parallel to the posterior digastric to insert in the hyoid.

Both the mylo-hyoid and the genio-hyoid muscles pull the hyoid bone and the tongue upward and forward and are very important in the initial stages of swallowing. Recent research shows intriguing new information about the genio-hyoid muscle. K. Honda suggests that this muscle, which has a direct insertion into the hyoid bone, is active at high frequencies in moving the hyoid bone forward, thus also rotating the thyroid forward and stretching the vocal folds. He calls this muscle "a supplementary tensor mechanism" and believes that it supplements crico-thyroid activity, especially for front vowels at higher frequencies.[13] Thus even though the genio-hyoid muscle is active in the beginning stages of swallowing, its activity may not be detrimental to all singing situations.

Secondary "false" elevators are the hyo-glossus (back of the tongue to the hyoid) and the genio-glossus (under the surface of the tongue to the hyoid). Studies by Honda and Baer

(1981) and Honda and Fujimura (1991) indicate that the posterior fibers of the genio-glossus raise the tongue dorsum (middle of the tongue) by drawing the tongue root forward on front vowels. The hyoid bone is moved forward and slightly downward, the thyroid cartilage rotates forward, and the vocal folds are stretched, an action similar to that of the genio-hyoid mentioned above. In contrast, the hyoid bone is moved up and backward on such low back vowels as /ɑ/ because of the retracted position of the tongue.[14] Contraction of the genio-glossus also widens the pharyngeal cavity, especially on very

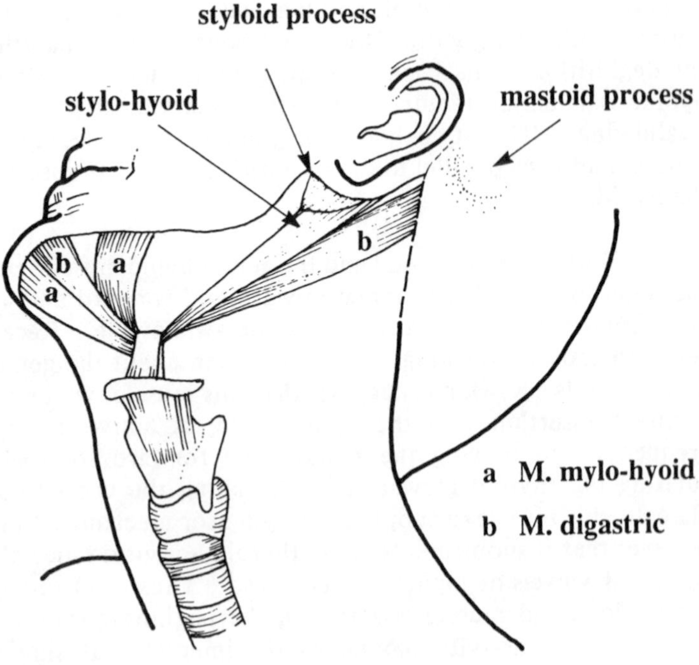

Fig. 16 Diagram of the False Elevators
Genio-hyoid is hidden by the mylo-hyoid.

high pitches, and the front of the pharyngeal wall shifts forward.[15] It would seem that another one of the "false" elevators has a positive rather than a negative influence upon cavity coupling for certain kinds of voices and at certain frequencies. Further research is needed.

For the most part, however, the supra-hyoid elevators must be deactivated if undue functional tension is to be avoided. Relaxation of the upper neck area and the tongue muscles is the goal of every successful singing technique.

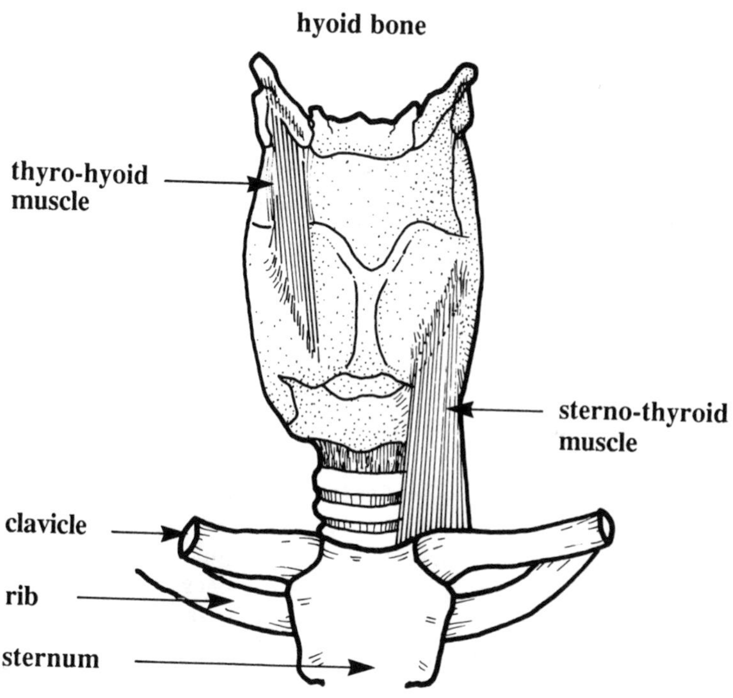

Fig. 17 Diagram of the primary antagonistic extrinsic muscles, the sterno-thyroid depressor and the thyro-hyoid elevator

If one considers the extrinsic musculature as a functional unit, muscular equilibrium is helpful in deactivating the "false" elevators. The hyoid bone continues to play a pivotal role in describing muscle function. Because it is so closely connected to the thyroid cartilage, the action of the hyoid determines in large measure the positioning of the larynx as a whole. Since the larynx is a flexible, floating structure, it is essential then that the elevator (upward) and the depressor (downward) muscles act as a unit, via muscular antagonism, and never independently. Proper use of this system is a prerequisite for optimum phonation and resonation, both of which are influenced by laryngeal positioning.

The Depressors

The depressors are those muscles that draw the larynx down and suspend it in a muscular sling from below.

The primary depressor is the paired sterno-thyroid which originates in the sternum and inserts in the sides of the thyroid cartilage. Its chief antagonists are the thyro-hyoid elevator and the crico-thyroid stretcher.

Secondary depressors include (see Fig. 18 for schematic line drawing):

(1) **Sterno-hyoid**. Originates in the sternum and inserts in the hyoid bone.

(2) **Omo-hyoid**. Originates on the upper border of the scapula or shoulder bone, passes through a loop arising from the collarbone, and inserts in the hyoid bone. A double-bellied muscle.

(3) **Crico-pharyngeal**. Originates from both lower sides of the cricoid and encircles the gullet at the junction of the pharynx and the esophagus. May widen the lower pharynx. The least developed of the entire network and the last to mature.

(4) **Trachea.** Exerts gravitational pull. Particularly evident as the diaphragm lowers on a deep breath.

It should be noted here that much more research needs to be done on the functioning of the crico-pharyngeal muscle. Saunders[16] feels that it "may pull the cricoid posteriorly, acting with the lateral crico-thyroid to stretch the cords" and Sonninen says the crico-pharyngeal anchors the cricoid.[17] Shipp believes "the downward pulling force of the crico-pharyngeous may facilitate the cricoid cartilage in its rocking action,"[18] thereby providing help in stretching the cords. Luchsinger takes an opposing view when he cites a Zenker study (1960) indicating that the crico-pharyngeal works antagonistically with the crico-thyroid to **shorten** the cords.[19] In the absence of irrefutable evidence one way or the other, we must rely upon empirical observation pending further research. Visual and aural evidence indicates that as the voice matures, the neck tends to jut forward if this muscle, together with the trapezius of the upper back, is not working. Often muscles of the tongue try to compensate for inaction of these important muscles.

The Elevators

As mentioned earlier, most of the "false" elevators are enemies of functional freedom and must be deactivated. The paired thyro-hyoid muscle, however, is seen as a superior extension of the primary depressor, sterno-thyroid. Certainly the two are major antagonists in this suspensory system. We shall call the thyro-hyoid the primary elevator. It originates in the side of the thyroid cartilage and inserts in the lower border of the hyoid. It is located beneath the omo-hyoid and the sterno-hyoid secondary depressors. When the thyroid cartilage is stable, i.e., anchored from below by the muscular pulleys of the sterno-thyroid muscles and the gravitational pull of the trachea, the thyro-hyoid and the hyoid bone also assume a stable position. A muscular equilibrium is achieved.

If, on the other hand, the hyoid is fixed in an elevated position and the depressors do not function, the thyroid cartilage and with it the entire larynx is excessively elevated. These major antagonists are shown in the diagram below and in Fig. 19.

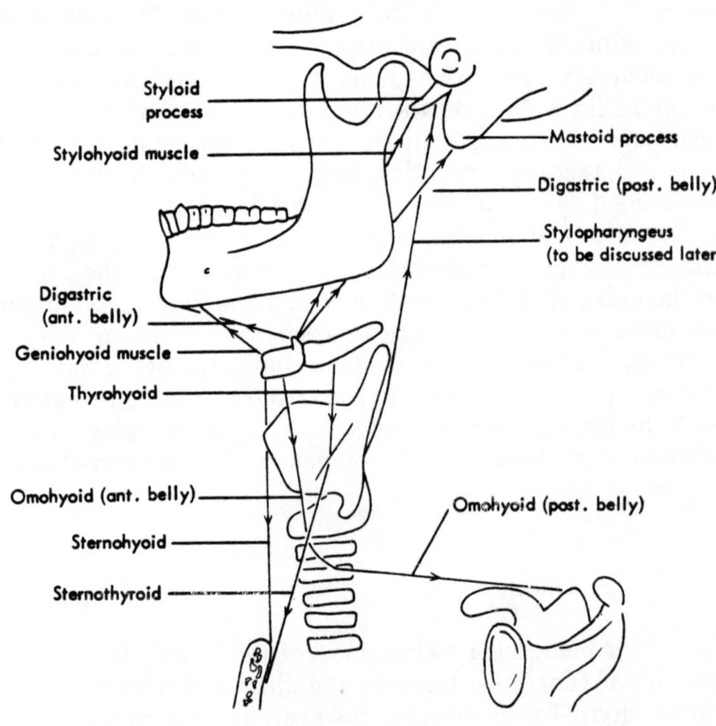

Fig. 18 Schematic of the actions of the extrinsic laryngeal muscles

Willard R. Zemlin, *Speech and Hearing Science: Anatomy & Physiology*, 3rd ed., 1988, p. 125. Reprinted by permission of Prentice-Hall, Inc., Englewood Cliffs, New Jersey.

The stylo-pharyngeal, a long muscle complex, arises from the styloid process, a bone which projects from the base of the skull just behind the jaw bone. Its fibers blend with the palato-pharyngeal to form a common muscle plate before ultimately inserting inside the top horn of the thyroid cartilage. As further evidence of the complex inter-relationships of this group of muscles, it is instructive to note that a section of the palato-pharyngeal muscle (also called pharyngopalatine) forms the posterior palatine arches (See the section on the soft palate in Chapter 6). Contraction of the stylo-pharyngeal network probably dilates the pharynx laterally. Certainly it tilts the thyroid cartilage forward to a maximal extent and thus moves the notch of the thyroid forward. Zenker (1960) indicates that this action can approximate the horns of the thyroid by as much as one centimeter, which undoubtedly accounts for the additional forward movement of the thyroid notch.[20] This action occurs most markedly at the transition from falsetto to head register and when dynamic levels go from soft to loud. At any rate, both glottal closure and vocal cord elongation are affected, particularly during loud high tones.

The stylo-pharyngeal is a secondary elevator, but is certainly not of secondary importance. When it works cooperatively with the crico-thyroid stretcher and is anchored by the contraction of secondary depressors, maximal longitudinal tension is produced in the vocal folds.

Zemlin says that contraction of this muscle group also "results not only in elevation of the pharynx but also in dilation."[21] Could this action be related to the lift feeling so necessary for top voice singing? If this secondary elevator is not synergistically activated, is soft palate action inadequate or muscular rigidity the result? These questions arise from subjective conjecture, but certainly introduce areas worthy of consideration and experimentation.

We definitely must conclude, however, based on laboratory investigation and on both aural and visual observation that use of the stylo-pharyngeal system is essential for optimal high voice production. Its use or lack of use has a major effect on phonation and on resonation.

Earlier in this chapter we talked about the composition of the major laryngeal cartilages and about some of the properties of hyaline. The thyroid cartilage may calcify or even ossify with age. Just as there are great individual differences in the onset of bone loss or osteoporosis, there is also great variation in the time and degree of ossification.

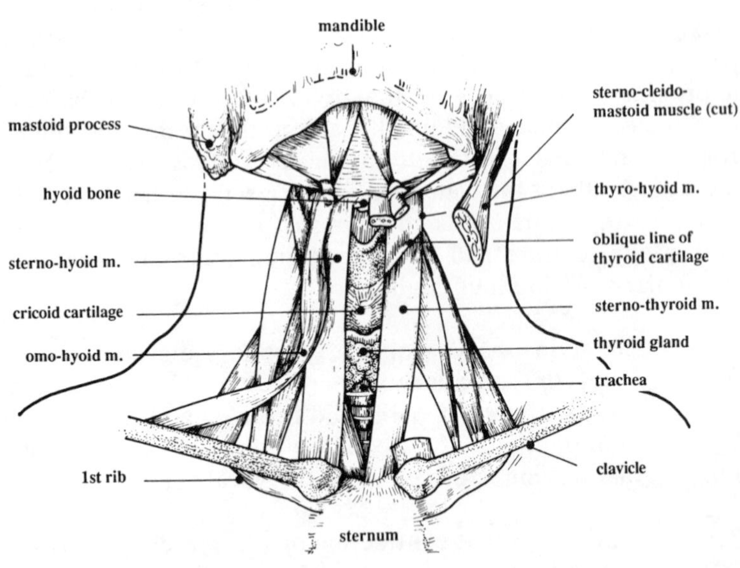

Fig. 19 Extrinsic muscles of the larynx

Although the aging voice generally struggles with deteriorating vocal quality and a marked decrease in agility, the most noticeable change is progressive loss of the top voice. As the thyroid horns calcify and eventually ossify, they are not flexible enough to be moved by contraction of the stylo-pharyngeal muscles.[22] The vocal folds lose glottal firmness and the ability to lengthen to their maximum. The top voice suffers. A more detailed review of recent studies on the aging voice is included in the appendix.

It should be noted here that there is a special danger for any singer who undergoes surgical removal of the thyroid gland. This important part of the endocrine system consists of two lobes, one on either side of the larynx. Sonninen (1956) reported on 76 patients with an age range of 15 to 70 years who had had thyroidectomies. Recovery was good if care had been taken not to cut the extrinsic muscles in front of the trachea. If these muscles were cut, voice range was impaired, particularly the top voice.[23]

Benefits of Extrinsic Equilibrium

Although the use of so many unfamiliar anatomical names may produce terminal jargonitis, an understanding of the part each of these muscles plays in the suspensory mechanism cannot be overemphasized. If the sterno-thyroid primary depressor works antagonistically with the thyro-hyoid primary elevator, the larynx stays in a steady, median position. As a result, the space in the pharynx is increased and undesirable tongue tension avoided. Cooperation between the sterno-thyroid and the crico-thyroid helps the latter stretch the vocal folds more gently and efficiently. The stylo-pharyngeal system, working on the horns of the thyroid cartilage, stretches the cords further for high voice singing, and this same system contributes to the widening of the pharyngeal cavity.

A moderately low, stable laryngeal position is essential for efficient vocal fold function and for the pharyngeal space needed in the full head voice. What happens, though, when the larynx is unduly depressed? The extrinsic muscles, particularly the depressors, are over-worked (hyperfunctional). Surprisingly, the intrinsic muscles are equally over-worked. Generally the head is also tipped forward so that the jaw is pressed into the larynx. In this position the vocalis and the lateral crico-arytenoid muscles are extremely hyperfunctional. There is very little increase in loudness, however, even though the vocalis is so active, and the tone sounds swallowed.[24] In a strained, pinched production, on the other hand, when the larynx is too high, the intrinsic muscles are over-worked, while the extrinsic network is under-worked (hypofunctional).

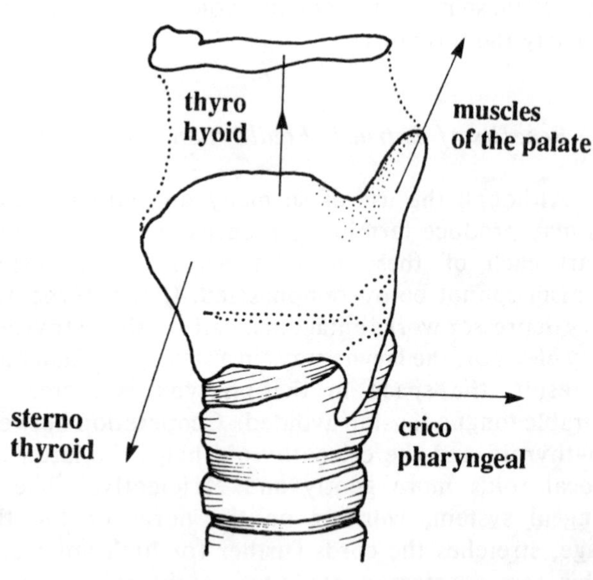

Fig. 20 Directional Schematic of the Suspensory Network

Inactivity of the suspensory mechanism results in poor coordination between the larynx and the breathing apparatus. The head and neck jut forward, air under too much pressure pushes against the cords, and the pharyngeal cavity is in a squeezed, tight configuration. Even the most musical singer cannot sing a flowing line if the vocal organ is poorly coordinated. It is also probable that until the suspensory muscles are properly developed and balanced, accurate voice classification is impossible.

NOTES

1. These two folds stretch from the upper tips of the arytenoid cartilages to the epiglottis, thus forming the lateral boundaries of the laryngo-pharynx. The cuneiform cartilages are small cone-shaped cartilages embedded in the aryepiglottic folds. Their importance will be discussed in more detail in the section on the singing formant in Chapter 6.

2. Willard R. Zemlin, "Notes on the Morphology of the Human Larynx: A Tutorial," *NATS Bulletin*, 41:1 (1984), 6.

3. Ingo Titze, "Sources of Irregularity in Vocal Fold Vibration," *NATS Journal*, 45:1 (1988), 23.

4. Zemlin, *Speech and Hearing*, op. cit., 108.

5. Appelman, op. cit., 79.

6. William H. Saunders, *The Larynx* (Summit, N.J.: CIBA Pharmaceutical Co., 1964), p. 41; W. J. Gould, "Effect of Respiratory and Postural Mechanisms upon Action of the Vocal Cords," *Folia Phoniatrica*, 23 (1971), 222; and Luchsinger and Arnold, op. cit., 73.

7. Manuel Garcia, *Hints on Singing* (London: Ascherberg, Hopwood & Crew, 1894), 6.

8. Cited in Luchsinger and Arnold, op. cit., 75.

9. Minoru Hirano, "Vocal Mechanisms in Singing: Laryngeal and Phoniatric Aspects," *Journal of Voice*, 2:1 (1988), 57.

10. William Vennard, *Singing: The Mechanism and the Technic*, Fourth ed. (New York: Carl Fischer, 1967), 63.

11. 1968 Sonninen research (Ann NY Acad Sci 155: 68-90) cited by Stella Hertegard, Jan Gauffin, and Johan Sundberg, "Open and Covered Singing as Studied by Means of Fiberoptics, Inverse Filtering, and Spectral Analysis," *Journal of Voice*, 4:3 (1990), 220-230.

12. William Vennard, "Some Implications of the Sonninen Research," *NATS Bulletin*, 15:4 (1959), 13.

13. Kiyoshi Honda and Osamu Fujimura, "Intrinsic Vowel F^0 and Phrase-Final F^0 Lowering: Phonological vs. Biological Explanations," Chapter 19, Jan Gauffin and Britta Hammarberg, eds., *Vocal Fold Physiology* (San Diego: Singular Publishing Group, 1991), 149-157.

14. Honda and Fujimura, ibid., 149. See also Kiyoshi Honda and Thomas Baer, "External Frame Function, Pitch Control, and Vowel Production," *Care of the Professional Voice.* Transcripts of the Tenth Symposium, Part I, Van Lawrence, ed. (New York: The Voice Foundation, 1981), 67; and Maureen Stone, Kathleen A. Morrish, Barbara C. Sonies, Thomas H. Shawker, "Tongue Curvature: A

Model of Shape during Vowel Production," *Folia Phoniatrica*, 39 (1987), 308.

15. Honda and Baer, op. cit., 67.

16. Saunders, op. cit., 44.

17. Cited in Vennard, "Sonninen Research," op. cit., 76.

18. Thomas Shipp, "Vertical Laryngeal Position in Singing," *Journal of Research in Singing*, 1:1 (1977), 19.

19. Cited in Luchsinger and Arnold, op. cit., 76.

20. Ibid., 76.

21. Zemlin, *Speech and Hearing*, op. cit., 275.

22. Joel C. Kahane, "Age Related Histological Changes in the Human Male and Female Laryngeal Cartilages: Biological and Functional Implications," *Care of the Professional Voice.* Transcripts of the Ninth Symposium, Part I, Van Lawrence, ed. (New York: The Voice Foundation, 1980), 15.

23. Vennard, "Sonninen Research," op. cit., 9-13.

24. William Vennard and Minoru Hirano, "Varieties of Voice Production," *NATS Bulletin*, 27:3 (1971), 27-28.

Chapter 3

PHONATION

The concept of making a sound is a simple operation, but in practice it is as complex as any task performed by the human body. We have discussed the cyclical process of breathing and the musculature of the larynx and its adjoining areas. Now we come to the coordination of the motor (breath) and the vibrator (vocal folds). The function of the resonators will be examined in a later chapter.

There can be no question that delicate and precise muscular adjustments are necessary to acquire the desired equilibrium of functions. In the act of phonation the primary task of the singer is to achieve the most efficient balance between the air stream and the tension in the muscles of the vibrator.

Phonation is the act of making a sound. In the interests of clarity of terminology, it is not the same as phonetics. Phonetics means the study and systematic classification of speech sounds, although its popular connotation refers to the pronunciation and articulation of words.

The anatomy of the vocal cords was described in some detail in the preceding chapter. Considering their amazing strength and resilience, they are surprisingly small muscles. They vary in length from 7/8 inch in low male voices to 3/8 inch in children and only 1/8 inch in infants. The vocal stamina and projection of a baby's cry are a testament to optimum function.

As the vocal folds begin to come together, the pressure of the subglottic air (beneath the folds) rises and the speed as its flow through the glottal passage increases. It is estimated that if the glottal chink is narrowed to about three millimeters, a very small amount of air flow is sufficient to set the folds into vibration.[1] This effect of air flow on the cords can be explained by an aerodynamic law called the Bernoulli effect. When a gas is in motion, it exerts less than its normal pressure upon its surrounding environment.[2] Stated another way, "when there is increased motion of gas molecules, there will be decreased pressure."[3] Air is a gas. Thus when the vocal lips are close enough to each other, the air moves at greater speed because of the narrowing of the glottal chink. The result is a reduced or negative pressure between the edges of the folds, and they are literally sucked together. There is a simple way to illustrate the Bernoulli effect. Take two sheets of paper and while holding them slightly apart, blow gently into the area between them. The sheets of paper will be pulled together. The normal atmospheric pressure on the outside surfaces of each sheet is greater than the moving air being blown between them; the velocity of the air increases and the pressure decreases.

To this aerodynamic action must be added the myoelastic (muscular) one. When the vocal folds are closed, they hold back the air stream until the subglottic air pressure becomes greater than their tension. Then a tiny puff of air escapes, reducing the pressure until cordal closure stops the flow of air again.

Phonation is a myoelastic-aerodynamic phenomenon. Highspeed pictures (4,000 frames per second) show a vocal fold vibratory pattern which emphasizes aerodynamic factors. Although the muscular element is present, the old concept that muscle tension versus breath pressure gives the whole picture is no longer accepted. Visual evidence has even confirmed that frequently the muscular or front portions of the folds are sucked together much more rapidly than the arytenoid cartilages can approximate the cartilaginous or back section.[4] Although the difference between these two approaches to vocal onset may be seen and studied only through high-speed pictures because the oscillatory speed of the cords is so fast, differences in the resulting tone can easily be heard by a discriminating ear. Brass players describe the aerodynamic approach as the "sweet" attack and the myoelastic one as the "buzz" attack.

The sequence of events for the simultaneous or "sweet" attack is:

(1) flow of breath sucks the glottis closed
(2) flow stops until breath pressure blows the glottis open
(3) air flow begins again and the cycle is repeated

For A^4 at 440 cycles per second the progression just described takes place 440 times per second. The two factors of the adductors closing the glottis and the air flowing must occur simultaneously to achieve the perfect attack. The glottis opens up and closes down once during a single cycle of vibration. These two actions are called adduction (bringing together) and abduction (moving apart).

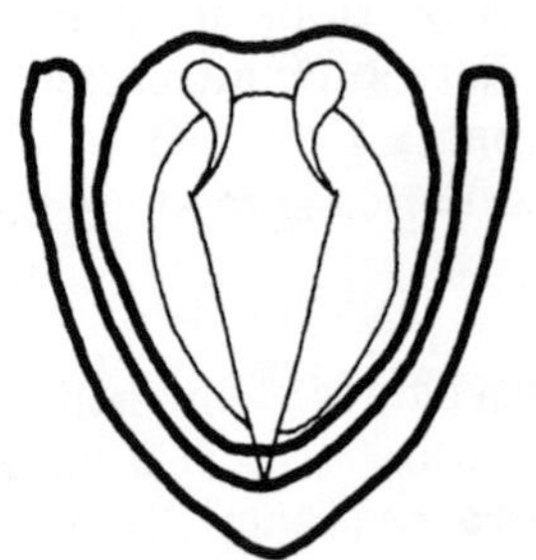

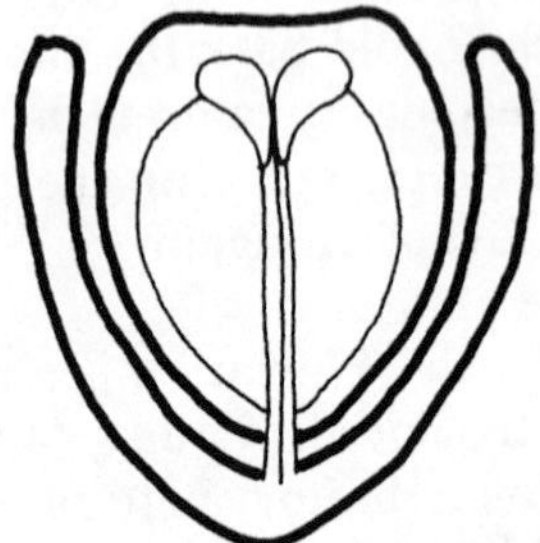

Fig. 21 Abduction and Adduction of the Vocal Folds

Looking down on the vocal folds in Fig. 21, the right figure shows them adducted. In the left diagram they are abducted for quiet breathing. During heavy, fast breathing (not shown), they are bowed out so that more air can pass through the glottis.

There are two kinds of phonation which should be avoided. If the breath is flowing before approximation of the vocal folds, a loosening of the valve takes place prior to phonation, and the tone begins with a breathy sound which disappears as full adduction is reached. This kind of attack is rare in adults; breathiness is more commonly caused by poor breathing and/or inefficient resonation. Regardless of the aesthetic questions involved, an aspirate attack is not vocally destructive, merely an inefficient kind of voice production.

The glottal plosive **is** destructive, however, and may lead to vocal nodules (small calluses on the cords). In the hard glottal attack, the arytenoids are brought together sharply and then breath pressure is applied to overcome the muscular tension. The degree of muscular tension generally determines how damaging the process is. A glottal plosive is similar to a slight cough; it is not vocally healthy and may eventually cause damage in some larynxes. If, however, the arytenoids are slammed together and the air hits the cords with an audible pop, the damage is much more severe and can happen in a very short time. Under these conditions the larynx is extremely constricted and elevated in the throat, the arytenoids are pressed together tightly, and a sizable number of vibratory cycles may take place before the muscular portion of the vocal folds begins to vibrate at all (this "hard" glottal attack is prevalent in some kinds of rock singing, in cheerleading, during shouting and screaming at sports events such as football or basketball games, or at noisy parties). Laryngologists confirm that this kind of phonation is extremely harmful, and all singing teachers and choral directors who understand what happens physically have an ethical obligation to discourage its use. Functional freedom of the singing instrument is impossible when it is used. The air is under excessive pressure, the vocal folds are being abused, the larynx is generally too high, the extrinsic musculature is collapsed, and the resonating cavities are tight and squeezed.

For high frequencies, the number of vibratory cycles increases and the cords generally become longer and tauter; the reverse is true for low frequencies. Another characteristic of low frequency vibration is called the vertical phase difference. The folds are thick, and the glottis closes at the bottom before it closes at the top, just as it opens at the bottom before it opens at the top. This action makes the folds look like waving flags, in contrast to almost no vertical phase difference at higher frequencies when the folds are thinner.

There is still controversy about what Manuel Garcia meant when he advocated the use of the ***coup de glotte***. Does the phrase mean stroke of the glottis or articulation of the glottis, a fine semantic point? It is interesting to note that Morell MacKenzie in 1890 saw no need to discuss the subject or to argue on one side or the other. He did disagree with Garcia on a number or pedagogical points, but apparently the ***coup de glotte*** was not one of them. Dr. MacKenzie says that "the ***coup de glotte***, or exact correspondence between the arrival of the air at the larynx and the adjustment of the cords to receive it is a point that cannot be too strongly insisted upon."[5] In any event, Garcia himself did warn against confusing the proper articulation with what he called the stroke of the chest, which resembles a cough.[6] Twentieth century technology has shown us what happens during a cough, and the glottal plosive is formed in the same way, although generally not so forcefully. In the aerodynamic-myoelastic attack, on the other hand, clean, precise articulation is the goal with no danger of the vibrator either being abused, being starved for air, or producing insufficient adductive pressure.

Subglottic pressure is the pressure just below the vocal folds and is the result of a complex system of breathing and phonatory factors. For very soft phonation, for instance, a low pressure of 3 cm H_2O is adequate and probably is primarily generated by the passive recoil of the lungs and of the intercostals. A pressure of about 20 cm H_20 is probably suffient for loud sounds, whether it be in singing or speaking, although as much as 70 cm H_20 is possible (although probably not desirable) under unusual singing conditions. In contrast, a subglottic pressure of up to 150 cm H_2O is possible during heavy lifting or for some brass instrument playing.[7]

Between the extremes of subglottic pressure/airflow ratios are many variations of "normal" phonation. On the one hand, singers consistently sing out of tune if they fail to use the proper subglottic pressure. You will note that we did not say a high subglottic pressure because the frequency of the sung sound is generally more crucial than dynamic changes.

> For arriving happily at a low note after a high one, it is necessary to reduce subglottal pressure appropriately. If the reduction is not great enough, subglottal pressure will be too high for the low note, and in extreme cases the folds may even fail to vibrate under such conditions.[8]

As in the case of the amount of air needed for the longest musical phrase (discussed in Chapter 1), there are great differences between individual singers. Too much pressure is probably more common than too little, especially considering the competitive personalities of most singers. In cases when a singer is running out of air, the temptation is great to decrease air flow and increase subglottic pressure. The appropriate ratio is then thrown out of balance, and a stiff, pressed sound results.

In a fascinating article on glottal aerodynamics in a recent issue of the *Journal of the Acoustical Society of America*, Ingo Titze states that singers get two to three times greater peak air flow for a given lung pressure than non-singers, and he hypothesizes that singers adjust their glottal or vocal tract configurations for optimum transfer between the vibrator and the resonator.[9] To obtain greater amplitudes of vibration for a given subglottic pressure, singers may be using additional thickening of the folds, a loosening adjustment of the vocal ligament, or greater air flow.

Factors that determine the fundamental frequency and the intensity of a sound are:

(1) Vocal fold tension or glottal resistance
(2) Aerodynamic power (ratio of subglottic pressure to air flow)
(3) Length of the vocal folds
(4) Mass of the vocal folds

At lower frequencies, pitch and intensity control are largely regulated by glottal resistance, the degree and closure time of the vocal folds themselves (determined primarily by the interaction of the vocalis and the crico-thyroid muscles). At higher frequencies, though, glottal resistance is no longer the major factor. Air flow is. This is not to say that air flow is the sole determinant of intensity at high frequencies. As early as 1965, a study showed that "the flow rate is not greatly affected" by greater intensity at low frequencies, but at high frequencies, the flow rate almost doubled (for both sexes) for a ten-decibel increase in vocal intensity.[10] Needless to say, the combinations of lung pressure and glottal resistance vary greatly with individual voices and singing techniques, and with a singer's physical condition, just as breathing techniques did in Chapter 1.

Gauffin and Sundberg (1989), propose the term "flow phonation" for a kind of production that has the highest possible air flow combined with complete glottal closure.[11] To those critics who may think that flow phonation advocates the use of too much air, the authors say "... it is often advocated that a generous airflow is advantageous for the vocal fold function."[12]

Titze concurs with Gauffin and Sundberg and sets forth his substantiating arguments in telling fashion.[13] Instead of the more commonly used factors listed earlier, he cites three kinds of adjustments that regulate vocal intensity.

(1) Below the larynx
(2) Within the larynx
(3) Above the larynx

Below the larynx, the aerodynamic power is a product of subglottic pressure and air flow. Within the larynx, this aerodynamic power is converted into acoustic power, and the control mechanism for this conversion is the pre-phonatory glottal width. The slight spreading of the vocal processes of the arytenoid cartilages during "flow phonation" is a sign of increased glottal width. How then does this regulation by glottal width compare with regulation by subglottic pressure? Titze says that if the pressure is held constant, acoustic power rises about 3 dB with a one-millimeter increase in glottal width, mainly because of increased flow.[14] He goes on to theorize that a 4-7 dB variation is possible via glottal width compared with an 8-9 dB increase by doubling subglottic pressure.[15] The former is preferred when speed of adjustment and fine control are needed. It also, for obvious reasons, produces less fatigue in the vocal fold musculature. Although many pedagogs favor a loud dynamic level at high frequencies rather than a slightly breathy sound, what price is paid for forceful, pressed phonation? In another recent study, "... professional tenors produced 10-12 dB greater intensity than nonsingers, primarily because their peak airflow was much higher for the same pressure."[16]

Because the "appropriate" ratio varies so much with combinations of pitch, intensity, vowel, register, and dynamic level, exact modes of behavior are difficult, if not impossible, to classify. "When the complexities of airway resistance generated by the articulators, coupled with the complexities of the laryngeal resistance ... are considered, the interactions between muscular effort, air flow, airway resistance, and subglottal pressure virtually defy description."[17] Singers and singing teachers do need to understand, though, that air flow and subglottic pressure are not the same, although they may work together to achieve the "sweet" attack. The paradoxical nature of these interactions is described by Dr. Wilbur J. Gould, co-chairman of *The Voice Foundation*.

> Although producing greater intensity would seem to require a greater effort, this increased

> effort is largely subjective, and the consciousness of the effort decreases, with training, until it almost appears that less effort is necessary.[18]

In the classical pedagogical books of the 18th and 19th centuries, most of them written by legendary singing teachers, the concept of "singing on the breath" recurs again and again. Even without scientific evidence such as we have today, they heard and recognized the perfect attack and the appropriate aerodynamic power needed, and they attempted to describe what they had heard. "Singing on the breath" is an ideal illustration of the empirical approach of these master teachers. There is much to be learned from a careful study of their writings because the basic methodology of western classical singing is reflected in their pedagogical concepts.[19]

It seems desirable, in light of the aerodynamic-myoelastic nature of phonation, to emphasize breath flow rather than excessive muscular pressure. Too much air flow probably is preferable to and certainly is less damaging than not enough. Optimum phonation occurs when subglottic pressure is the result of ample air flow and firm closure of the cords. On the other hand, subglottic pressure produced by trying to rectify inadequate air flow through excess abdominal muscular pressure is probably as inefficient and potentially injurious as excessive muscular tension of the vocal folds.

It clearly is much easier to define what should not be done than to devise a method of breathing that will work for all singers. The only real consensus is that a combination of abdominal (or diaphragmatic) and thoracic breathing encourages the best cooperation between the air stream and the vibrating vocal folds.

NOTES

1. Zemlin, *Speech and Hearing*, op. cit., 144.

2. Vennard, *Singing*, op. cit., 39.

3. Raymond H. Colton and Janina K. Casper, *Understanding Voice Problems* (Baltimore: Williams and Wilkins, 1990), 286.

4. Vennard, "The Bernoulli Effect in Singing," *NATS Bulletin*, 17:3 (1961), 10.

5. Morell MacKenzie, *Hygiene of the Vocal Organs* (London: Macmillan, 1890), 110.

6. Manuel Garcia, *The Art of Singing*, Part I (Boston: Oliver Ditson, ca. 1855), 11.

7. R. Leanderson and J. Sundberg, "Breathing for Singing," *Journal of Voice*, 2:1 (1988), 4.

8. Ibid., 10.

9. Ingo Titze, "Phonation Threshold Pressure: A Missing Link in Glottal Aerodynamics," *Journal of the Acoustical Society of America*, 91:5 (1992), 2926-2935.

10. N. Isshiki, "Vocal Intensity and Air Flow Rate," *Folia Phoniatrica*, 17:2 (1965), 92-104.

11. Jan Gauffin and Johan Sundberg, "Spectral Correlates of Glottal Voice Source Waveform Characteristics," *Journal of Speech and Hearing Research*, 32:3 (1989), 559.

12. Ibid., 563.

13. Ingo R. Titze, "Regulation of Vocal Power and Efficiency by Subglottal Pressure and Glottal Width," Chapter 19, *Vocal Fold Physiology: Voice Production, Mechanisms and Functions*, Osamu Fujimura, ed. (New York: Raven Press, 1988), 227-238.

14. Ibid., 236.

15. Ibid., 237.

16. Ingo R. Titze and Johan Sundberg, "Vocal Intensity in Speakers and Singers," *Journal of the Acoustical Society of America*, 91:5 (1992), 2936.

17. Zemlin, *Speech and Hearing*, op. cit., 92.

18. W. J. Gould, "The Pulmonary-Laryngeal System," Chapter 3, *Vocal Fold Physiology*, K. N. Stevens and M. Hirano, eds. (Tokyo: University of Tokyo Press, 1981), 26.

19. Berton Coffin, *Historical Vocal Pedagogy Classics* (Metuchen, N.J.: Scarecrow Press, 1989. Reprints of 18 articles originally published in *NATS Bulletin* between 1981 and 1984).

Chapter 4

POSTURE

Almost all pedagogical books dealing with the physiology of the singing instrument talk about posture and breathing first, in that order. Why then are they separated here? Good posture certainly is an essential prerequisite for good breathing. No one will argue that point. It also has a very important, and sometimes overlooked effect, however, upon laryngeal positioning and phonation. Above the vocal folds the filtering and the projection of sound take place. Although muscular equilibrium and functional interdependence are mandatory for the entire vocal instrument, acoustical matters are of prime importance there. Consequently, it seems most appropriate for posture to be considered after phonation.

The singing voice is the only musical instrument that has its home inside the body, which makes how one holds that body of primary importance. While posture, breathing, and phonation form a complex system of balancing mechanisms, it is posture that determines the efficiency of the muscles that power the system. Posture is the common denominator. As a matter of fact, posture is a kinesthetic barometer for the entire body, continually giving us conceptual data on body position, muscle tone, energy potential, and balance. This data is received from the sensory nerves associated with the muscles. Thus the kinesthetic sense, although not one of the commonly acknowledged five senses, is the subtle regulator of the complicated body patterns of movement and rest. The interdependent relationship between the breathing and the phonatory mechanisms is fostered by kinesthetic awareness. An intriguing hypothesis is the idea that changes in breathing patterns may be a *result* of changes in posture. Certainly the effect of posture on laryngeal function is equally significant. "... when the gross posture is 'correct' and when the extrinsic muscles are active, then the intrinsic laryngeal muscles may be most relaxed or free to perform efficiently. ..."[1]

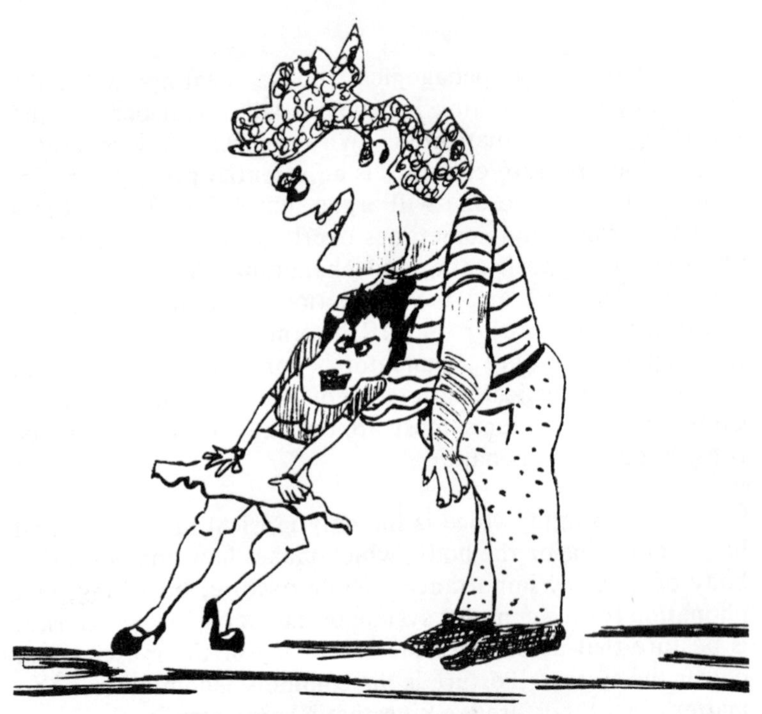

Stand Up!

The singer must be aware of his/her preparatory stance, that physical attitude of the body from which athletes start their particular activities. Like all athletes, individual singers have their own unique physical characteristics. A general picture can be drawn, however, of the kind of posture needed. Basic to achieving a dynamic, well-balanced skeletal alignment is the feeling of spinal stretch. If one imagines strings attached to the skull behind each ear and to the top of the sternum, like a puppet, the rest of the body does not have to be pushed and pulled into place in bits and pieces.

(1) The head is erect on the shoulders, not projected forward or pulled back.
(2) The chest is comfortably high with the rib cage in an open position.
(3) The shoulders are slightly back, but relaxed and down.
(4) The arms hang loosely at the sides and do not "invade" the chest area.
(5) The pelvis rests in a suspended position below the spread-out rib cage.
(6) Stand buoyantly as if ready for action. Do not put your weight on your heels, but balance directly above the arch of your foot to take advantage of this tiny trampoline.

The reason for the non-specific statement about the pelvic position is that it depends a great deal upon neck and rib cage alignment. If one bends over to touch the floor, it is easy to tell at what point the torso bends and where the actual hip joint is. Most hip joints are much lower than we imagine. Probably that is why bending from the waist is such hard work and so inefficient. When we find the exact location of the hip joint, alignment of the head, the open rib cage, and the pelvis is much easier. We are not trying to "put" this major joint where it is not. If a lengthening and stretching of the spine is felt, habitually compressed muscles will release so that we feel lightly balanced and almost weightless. Any undue pressure on vertebral discs is relieved and the position of the pelvis is then a natural, poised one. If, however, we try to keep the buttocks "tucked in," the gluteal muscles generally become very tense, and that tension is communicated to other parts of the torso and sometimes even to the knees.

There is almost as much controversy about where to position the feet as there is about whether to breathe through the mouth or the nose. In both instances, it depends upon the circumstances. From a kinesthetic point of view, it is best not to stand with the feet too close together because total body balance can too easily be compromised. Particularly detrimental to proper pelvic alignment is the stance advocated in beauty competitions. Not only are the legs and feet too close together, but the feet are angled out in a duck-like manner. The subject of such artificial posture looks as if she could be toppled by a light breeze. Other than this caveat, however, there is no need to be adamant about exactly where each foot is placed. If you check your appearance in a full length mirror from time to time, you will note that for certain songs you take a more assertive body position than for others, depending upon the dramatic intent of the words and music. After all, so-called "body language" should complement the color of the vocal sound, not divorce itself from any emotional involvement.

An open, preparatory, receptive posture is of great benefit to a singer's inner spirit, just as nervousness and fear produce a tense, destructive body set. After all, depression can be physical as well as emotional, and one state often brings about the other. The audience does not take long to sense the negative or positive non-verbal messages being sent. The physical evidence of a buoyant, receptive body is further enhanced by the open rib cage. A genuinely upright posture is seldom seen in today's society. Driving two blocks to the grocery store, sitting in front of the TV set an inordinate number of hours, using unsuitable furniture and carrying heavy book bags on one shoulder contribute to a tense body posture. No wonder so many people are in a slumped, drawn-in position most of the time.

The most common evidence of poor body alignment is a jutting chin and locked jaw plus a sunken chest and overly tight abdominal muscles. When an attempt is made to stand erect, many students feel as if they must surely fall over backwards. The chest in particular feels unduly exposed (as does the psyche). An upright position may feel abnormal at first, but practicing in front of a mirror will confirm how much better it looks and will reinforce this new way of standing and feeling. No one has stated the essence of this kind of posture better than the great Italian soprano of the turn of the century, Luisa Tetrazzini (1909).[2]

I have seen pupils, trying to master the art of breathing, holding themselves as rigidly as drum majors. Now this rigidity of the spinal column will in no way help you in the emission of tone, nor will it increase the breath control. In fact, I don't think it would even help you to stand up straight, although it would certainly give one a stiff appearance and one far removed from grace. A singer should stand freely and easily and should feel as if the chest were leading, but should not feel constrained or stiff in any part of the ribs or lungs.

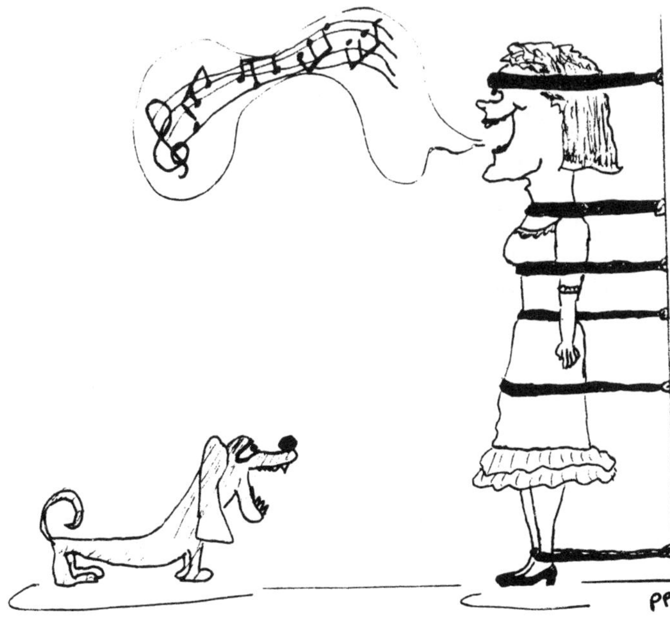

The Drum Majorette

Achieving a balanced relationship between the head, neck, and torso has received particular attention in recent years because of a growing interest in the Alexander Technique. F. M. Alexander, an Australian, was initially a singer and actor, but he had severe vocal problems. By trial and error, he found that the way in which we use ourselves physically affects how we function in every other area. The operative word here is "way." He believed that most of us are goal oriented and pay little or no attention to the way in which we attain those goals. Yet seemingly difficult tasks can be mastered not by trying harder, but by leaving the body alone to choose its own "position of mechanical advantage." He maintained that the body is capable of doing much more than imagined if we just stay out of its way. Of course, staying out of its way is more difficult to do than it sounds. Habitual misuse builds up over a long period of time, and bad habits come to feel familiar and right. We cannot even be sure we are doing what we think we are doing. Conceptual awareness becomes untrustworthy.

At the heart of the Alexander Technique is individual responsibility to consciously choose, the belief that inner freedom is expressed through self-discipline. Self-discipline begins with a desire to change inappropriate physical habits. Instead of doing what is habitual, one must consciously choose to act or not to act. By choosing not to act, one conceptually chooses to inhibit the undesirable habit. Alexander described the traditional way of dealing with incorrect habits. "We are taught to **do** something in order to correct it, instead of being taught, as a first principle, how to prevent (inhibition) the wrong thing from being done."[3] When one finally does act, the most important act is the next one, not the eventual goal of that specific exercise. It is apparent that Alexander's ideas are not limited to posture, although for him it was the outward manifestation of one's inner state.

Of all athletes, gymnasts provide the classic example of poise and balance. As they prepare to act, it is as if they are

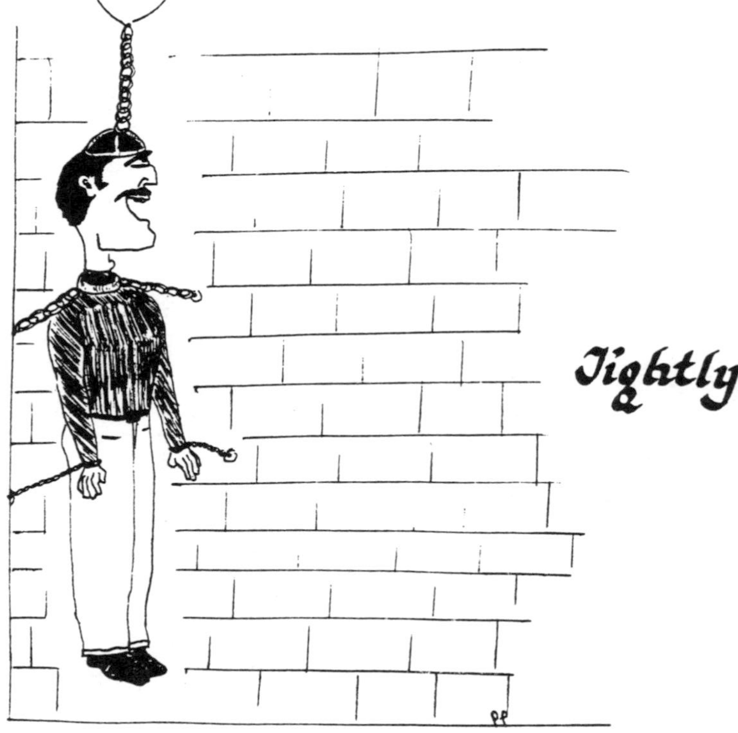

Tightly Coupled

observing themselves from a distance. They "listen" to themselves, to their kinesthetic barometers. There seems to be a delicate balance between control and spontaneity, and a noticeable lack of stiffness in the neck, shoulders, pelvis, and knees. The breath is not held back. Breathing is so slow and steady as to be unseen, and the graceful balance of the head on the shoulders is a characteristic of their sport. There are no hunched shoulders or pulled-in chins. A feeling of lightness and ease replaces unwanted muscular tension.

Stiffness and rigidity in the neck and shoulders are especially pervasive in our society. We are bombarded daily by a high level of sensory stimulation. A quiet atmosphere is a luxury, and unfortunately one which few people seek. Many people are not comfortable with silence. When a sedentary lifestyle is combined with constant sensory provocation, is it any wonder that too much body tension is so widespread and causes so many health problems?

Although the Alexander Technique advocates a "forward and up" position of the head, much depends upon what task is being undertaken. Alexander himself thought of the neck-head-shoulders relationship as a dynamic, ever-changing one and stated that there is no "right position." Some positions are more advantageous than others for specific tasks. No matter what position is taken, however, muscular tension in the neck must be released so that the back can lengthen and widen, and the chest can open up. A precise verbal formula is confining at best. It is interesting to note that Alexander's "primary movement," his early name for the primary requisite of good body use, is the greatest possible lengthening of the spine.[4]

The accuracy of the dictum of "forward and up" depends upon what is meant by forward. A head jutting too far forward throws the spine out of line and often is characteristic of a tense, over-achieving personality. On the other hand, if the head is drawn back and down, it compresses the spine, tucks the chin into the neck, and gives an overall

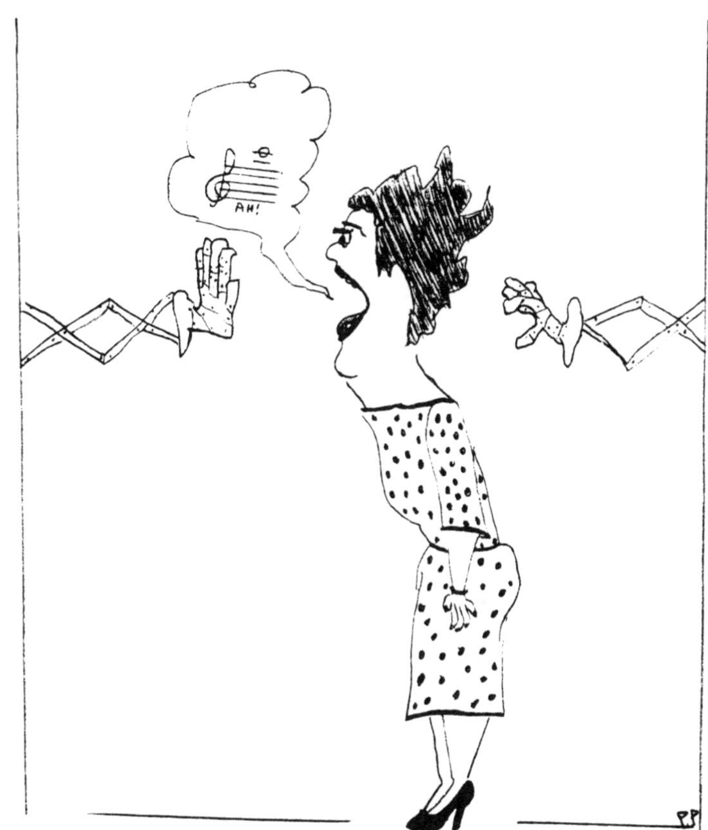

Eager Beaver

impression of a body being pulled down by gravity (both physically and figuratively). This position is unusually detrimental for singers because the extrinsic depressor muscles are overworked, optimum laryngeal positioning is at risk, and breathing is critically disturbed. If the head is down, the upper chest is allowed to drop, and the shoulders are rounded and tense as well. The cervical spine curves forward. Breathing becomes irregular and over-pressurized as the abdominal muscles use too much compensatory force and muscles in the jaw, neck, and tongue try to control the pressure. When the head is bowed, functional equilibrium of the suspensory network is sacrificed. The tone becomes too dark and lacks overtones; it will not carry. Like all parts of

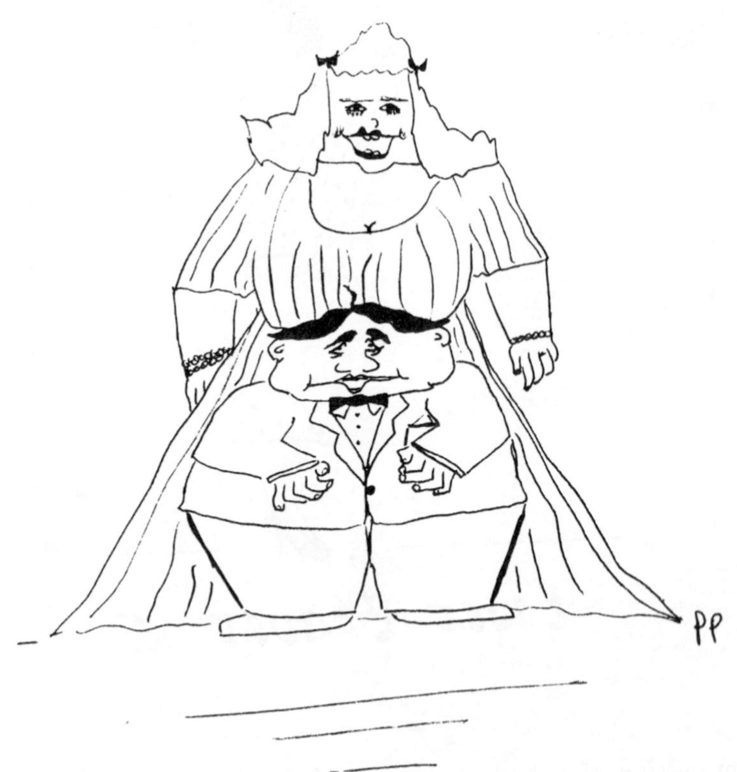

Keep your chest up!

the singing mechanism, the position of the larynx must be flexible and must be regulated primarily by head, neck, and respiratory factors. Immobility is an enemy of singing.

Just as the efficiency of a muscle is measured by its speed and mobility of action as well as its balance with other muscles rather than its sheer strength, so body posture is a matter of supple muscle tone and flexible balance. Body exercise needs to be carefully monitored in order to achieve suppleness and balance. Lifting excessively heavy weights sometimes creates more problems than it solves. Permanent shoulder and neck tension, restrictive compression of the spine, and the holding back of air are three of the more common consequences. Using light weights in exercises designed for specific flexibility and stretching purposes will build stamina without the risk of undesirable tension. Swimming, dancing, walking, and full-body exercise like racquet ball also are excellent body toning activities. Modern dance training is especially beneficial because it teaches fluid body movement, grace, and poise as well as providing a balanced muscular workout. It is an excellent way to replace ineffectual, random bobbing of the head and flailing of the arms with supple, genuinely "expressive" movements. Certainly dance training will wean the shy, distrustful singer from what Robert Edwin[5] calls the "fig leaf" position. Many young singers mistake such unmotivated, haphazard body movements for "communication" with an audience. On the contrary, uncontrolled, irrelevant body movement betrays a serious lack of kinesthetic and muscular stability. It is essential for both the singer and the singing teacher to realize that the most fundamental skill a singer must acquire is vocal production, not interpretive skills. "To reverse them is like a track coach emphasizing running strategy before teaching how to run."[6]

In the anticipatory, expectant stance advocated earlier, the head is up and tilted slightly. Observation of professional singers on TV confirms this position. It permits a balance between the upward and downward pulls of the muscles attached to the hyoid bone. In addition, there are muscles which pull the base of the skull downward slightly to elevate the head properly for singing. The sternomastoid and the trapezius, both postural muscles, are shown in Fig. 22. The sternomastoid also may help to elevate the upper chest.

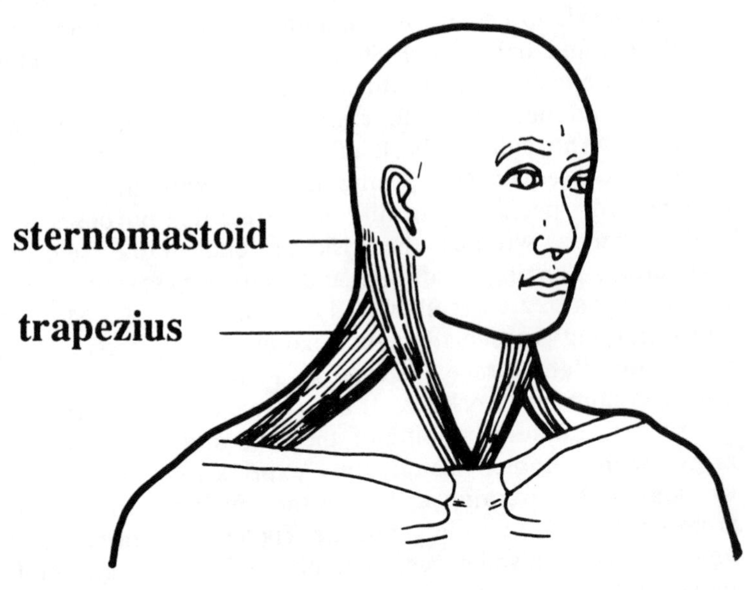

Fig. 22 Major Postural Muscles Affecting Head Position for Singing

For the top notes, the singer assumes a position unlike any other athlete. When describing a picture of Caruso singing a high note Beverley Johnson of the Juilliard School says:

> It shows him with his arms down, and his head back, and his jaw open, and you can see that he stands in an absolutely straight line.[7]

She goes on to say she also has found pictures of other famous singers, and for the high notes, this position is "almost a generality." The position is "akin to that of a sword swallower." Berton Coffin agrees with this assessment of head position for the top voice and shows a picture of Beniamino Gigli in that position.[8]

One of Alexander's aphorisms was that "feeling, when it is right, is of much more use than what they call mind."[9] A feeling of "up" signals anticipation, confidence, optimism. "Down" indicates depression and dejection. Thus the connotative meaning, what a word suggests, has both a physical and a mental effect on behavior. "Down" also means a depressed neck and spinal column and a dropped rib cage, whereas "up" brings about a balanced neck-torso bond, a lengthened and widened back, and an erect chest. The physical and the mental "feeling" merge.

The relationship between personal stress, poor posture, and lack of a reliable vocal technique is a close one. Singers are most often extroverts, and although they talk a lot, they do not necessarily talk about their personal problems. It is amazing also how many young people feel that physical difficulties are "legitimate," but that emotional problems are somehow their fault. It is not within the scope of this book to cover the psychological aspects of teaching singing, important as they are, but certainly a willingness to listen is an essential characteristic of any successful teacher and one of those many hats a teacher must wear.

Over and over, students say, "I feel as if I'm not working hard enough when I sing." Consequently, many of them oversing, using as much as ten times the amount of muscle energy needed. This inevitably leads to inaccurate mental concepts and inefficient physical habits. One of the many paradoxes in the art of singing is the maxim that "less is more." For the goal-oriented person, who believes that maximum effort is the key to success, this aphorism is particularly difficult to understand and to follow. Perhaps an

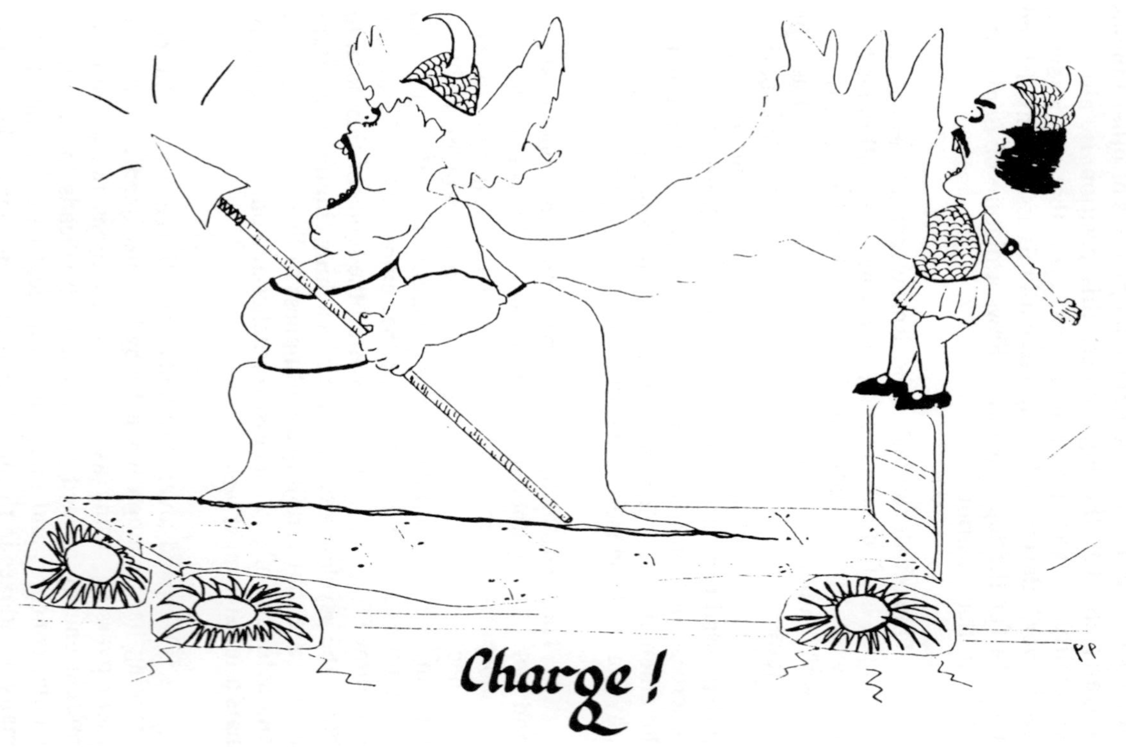
Charge!

alternate aphorism would be better understood: "relaxation is acquiring energy and freedom for action." The truly great performers and athletes show an ease and economy of resources that make their efforts look easy. This kind of relaxation can be learned, and at the base of such learning is kinesthetic awareness.

NOTES

1. Jo Estill, Thomas Baer, Kiyoshi Honda, and Katherine S. S. Harris, "An EMG Study of Supralaryngeal Activity in Six Voice Qualities," *Care of the Professional Voice*, Transcripts of the Thirteenth Symposium, Part 1, Van Lawrence, ed. (New York: The Voice Foundation, 1984), 67.

2. Enrico Caruso and Luisa Tetrazzini, *Caruso and Tetrazzini on the Art of Singing*. 1909 Reprint (New York: Dover Publications, 1975), 15.

3. From "Our Mistaken Ideas about Ourselves" contained in Edward Maisel, ed., *The Resurrection of the Body* (Writings of F. M. Alexander). (New York: Dell Publishing, 1969), 19.

4. Cited by Maisel, op. cit., xxiii, and identified as a statement by Alexander in 1907.

5. Robert Edwin, "The Language of the Body," *NATS Journal*, 48:4 (1992), 37.

6. Leon Thurman and Van Lawrence, "Voice Care for Vocal Athletes in Training," *The Choral Journal*, 20:9 (1980), 34.

7. Panel Discussion, "Update on Vocal Registers," *Care of the Professional Voice*, Transcript of the Eighth Symposium, Part I, Van Lawrence, ed. (New York: The Voice Foundation, 1979), 113.

8. Berton Coffin, *Overtones of Bel Canto* (Metuchen, NJ: Scarecrow Press, 1980), 179.

9. Quoted in Michael Gelb, *Body Learning: An Introduction to the Alexander Technique* (London: Aurum Press, 1983), 38.

Chapter 5

THE PHYSICAL NATURE OF SOUND

Characteristics of a Sound Wave

The life of sound begins in the vibrator (vocal folds), continues by transmission through an elastic medium (air), and is received by the ear of the hearer. From then on, the mind interprets the incoming data.

What is a sound wave and how does it move through air? It is no accident that physicists have chosen to call the products of a vibrator sound "waves." There is a certain similarity between the behavior of sound vibrations in air and waves in water. In both cases there is motion through a particular medium, either air or water, but the individual molecules themselves do not move perceptibly.

Sound waves are actually alterations in pressure which propel themselves through an elastic medium. That medium is most often air. As they move, these pressure waves or sound waves alternately expand and contract. Each particle of the wave passes on the energy within the sound wave to its neighboring air particle. The compression (increased pressure) **phase** of the wave moves through the air, leaving behind it a rarefaction (decreased pressure) phase. Like a moving field of grain, each spear (or air particle) has its own backward and forward swing. Similarly, the energy of sound is transmitted through air, each particle of air imparting energy to the next particle within an air mass, but without any perceptible motion of the mass as a whole.

Like the bob of a pendulum or the motion of a swing, the slowest speeds of a simple harmonic sound wave (sine wave) occur at its two extreme positions, while the maximum speed takes place at the median of its oscillation. The system moves most rapidly as it passes through its median position, slows up, reverses, and accelerates again to maximum speed as it passes the median position in the opposite direction.

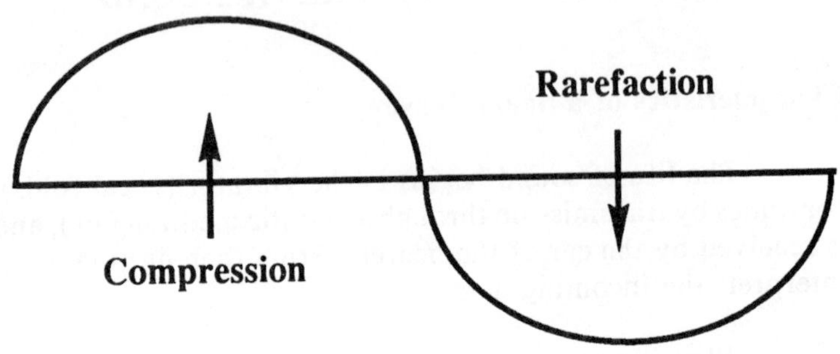

Fig. 23 A Simple Sine Wave

Properties of a Musical Sound

Acoustical and musical authorities agree that a musical sound possesses three distinct properties: frequency (pitch), amplitude (loudness), and timbre (tone quality).

Frequency

The concept of frequency was first proven in experiments by Marin Mersenne (1588-1648), the French physicist and musical theorist. Since that time, frequency has been defined as the number of vibratory cycles (one complete compression and rarefaction cycle) in one second, and is called cycles per second (cps) or Hertz (Hz). The time taken to complete one vibratory cycle is called the **period** of a sound wave. The period remains the same at a given frequency, and can be computed by dividing the speed of sound (approximately 1130 feet or 345 meters per second) by the frequency of the wave. For example, the wave length of A^4 is determined by dividing 1130 (the speed of sound) by 440 (the number of cycles per second) = about 2 1/2 feet. At the higher frequency of $F\sharp^5$ (740 cps), the same mathematical calculation yields a much shorter sound wave of approximately

1 1/2 feet. The higher the frequency, therefore, the greater the number of cycles per second and the shorter the sound wave. All sound, no matter what frequency, travels at the same speed through air.

Frequency (pitch) is varied by stretching, increasing the tension, and/or changing the mass of a vibrator. In the case of the singing voice, these factors are discussed in the chapter on registers.

Pitch is the mind's interpretation of frequency. The fluctuations in pitch standards during the various periods of music history substantiate the subjective nature of pitch. In Tudor times in England, church music was performed about a tone higher than it is today, while in 1751 Handel's tuning fork sounded about a half tone lower than today's official standard. This pitch of 422.5 for A^4 prevailed through the Beethoven period. It rose slightly toward the middle of the 19th century. Whenever Verdi found it climbing, for instance, he insisted on a return to 432 cps. One of his conditions for giving the Italian premiere of *Aida* to La Scala Opera was a return to proper pitch for A^4. Could he have had the soft high C at the end of "O Patria Mia" in mind? The pitch went up again when the brass instruments of the military band were developed in the second half of the 19th century. At the Vienna Opera in 1858, the pitch for A^4 was 456.1 cps. In 1939 an International Conference on Pitch was held in London and an "international pitch" of 440 cps for A^4 was decided upon. While the scientific world still holds to 426.6 cps, a frequency close to that of Handel's day, even the 440 figure has not held true in recent years. In the opera world, recent pitch inflation has reached as high as 460, much to the dismay of protesting singers who warn of vocal abuse and premature aging of young voices. Violin makers also are concerned about priceless old instruments that may not survive a tauter tuning.

In the area of 50 cps to 4,000 cps, the ear has maximum pitch and amplitude sensitivity. Subjective perception of amplitude does seem to decrease measurably below 1000 cps, and actual measured loudness levels in decibels are heard as much softer than at a higher frequency.[1] At the same time, high dynamic levels at low frequencies, generally below 1000 cps, produce lower subjective estimates of pitch, while at higher frequencies the opposite phenomenon occurs.[2] These phenomena are much more pronounced in relatively simple harmonic tones, however, than in more complex ones. At middle frequencies, pitch and loudness seem to be independent factors.

Amplitude

Amplitude, the second property of a musical sound, is the distance that a vibrator moves as it vibrates. Put another way, it is the amount of displacement of the vibrator from its rest position. In this case the vibrator is the vocal folds. A force (the air) is applied to the vocal folds, and a wave of a certain amplitude is produced. The larger the amplitude of vibration, the more intense the sound wave produced.

Most musical instruments are "transformers", i.e., they convert energy or power into audible sound. Most of this power is used to overcome friction. For instance, a large pipe organ requires a motor which generates 10,000 watts of power in order to blow it, but only 12 to 14 watts appear as sound. A pianist may use energy at the rate of 200 watts in a fortissimo passage with only four-tenths of a watt being radiated as sound. The human voice, on the other hand, is one of the most efficient transformers, although only about one percent of a singer's energies generally is converted into actual sound.[3]

The subjective evaluation by the ear of a sound's amplitude is called its loudness or intensity, although there is evidence that tone quality also has a bearing on intensity. It is often noted that high tones seem to have more intensity than low tones of the same amplitude, but again, the evaluation is probably influenced by the tone quality as well as the amplitude. It should be noted here that the average male larynx is on average about 20% larger than the female larynx. The vibrating portion of male vocal folds, therefore, is proportionately longer, and can drive more air and produce a larger amplitude of vibration.[4] On the other hand, female singers, as mentioned above, have the acoustical advantage of singing at higher frequencies.

Please refer to the definition of **phase** in the third paragraph of this chapter. Let us consider several examples of simple sine waves, all with the same period, but with varying amplitudes and/or phase patterns.

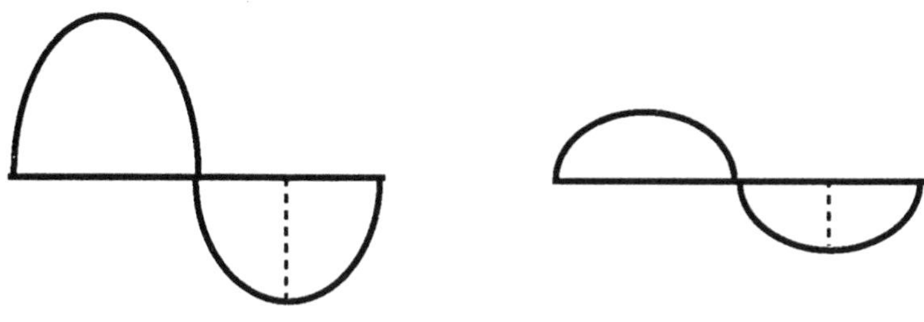

Fig. 24 Two Sine Waves with the same period
but different amplitudes
(amplitude indicated by dotted lines)

If the waves are of different amplitudes, but completely in phase, the resulting waveform has greater amplitude than either of its components (Fig. 25). If two waves of different amplitudes are completely out of phase or "out of step," however, the resulting wave has an amplitude smaller than that of the smaller of the two waves. Partial interference has taken place, and the amplitude of the sound has been seriously reduced (Fig. 26).

When two simple sine waves of the same amplitude come to a state of complete opposition of phase, an acoustical phenomenon known as total interference occurs. There is no sound at all. Although such an occurrence is rare for singers,

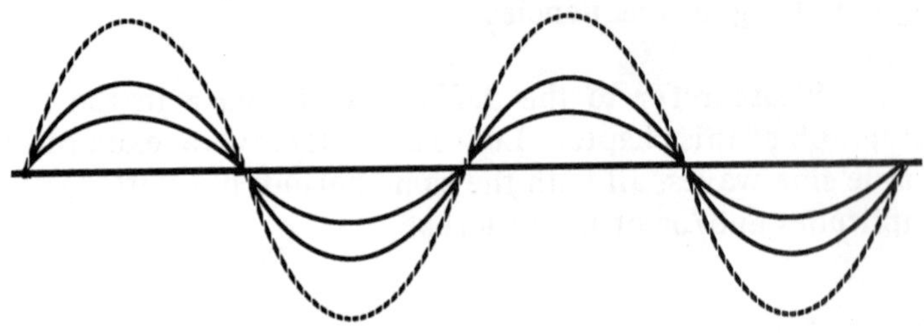

Fig. 25 Two sine waves of different amplitudes completely in phase (amplitude of resulting wave indicated by dotted line)

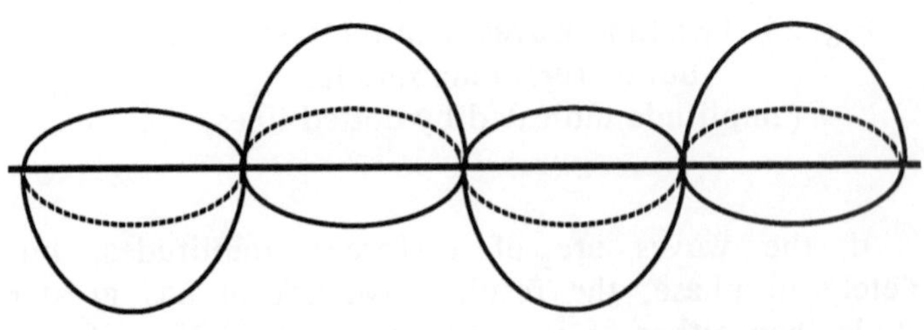

Fig. 26 Two sine waves of different amplitudes completely out of phase (amplitude of resulting wave indicated by dotted line)

it can happen, and should be treated as a resonance or acoustical problem, not a phonatory one (Fig. 27). Conversely, if the same two waves are totally in phase, the resultant waveform has twice the amplitude of either of its components. Obviously, this condition provides optimum intensity and projection.

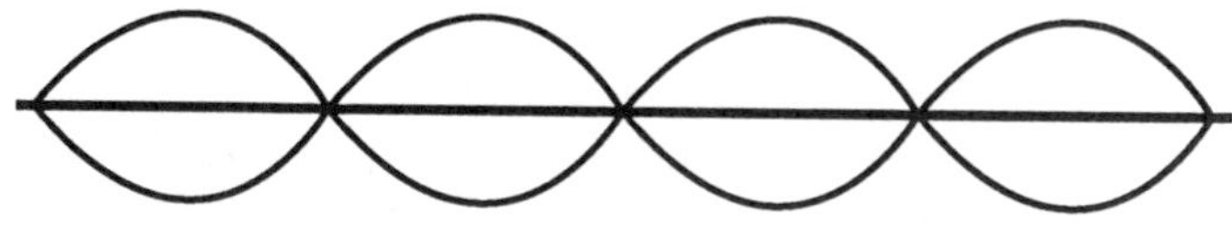

Fig. 27 Two sine waves of the same amplitude completely out of phase, producing no sound

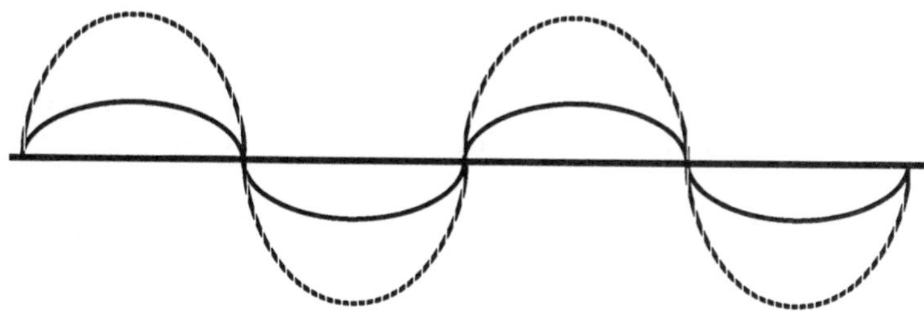

Fig. 28 Two sine waves of the same amplitude completely in phase (amplitude of resulting wave indicated by dotted line)

Timbre

The third major property of a musical sound, and perhaps the most distinguishing one, is timbre or tone quality. Quality is that characteristic which distinguishes a specific sound from the sounds of other voices or instruments, even though all the sounds are of the same fundamental frequency and amplitude. For example, timbre makes the difference between the sounds of a violin and those of an oboe, even though both tones may have the same frequency and intensity.

Thus far we have described sound waves which produce simple harmonic patterns such as those resulting from the vibrations of a tuning fork. Such simple sine wave patterns are unusual in the world of music; most sounds are the result of many simultaneous simple vibrations.

The sound of a clarinet playing A^4 is distinguished from any other musical sound of like frequency and amplitude because of the completely individualistic character of its pattern of vibrations. In 1800 J. B. Fourier, the French mathematician, showed that it is possible to break down any complex periodic vibration into a series of simple periodic motions, and further, that the frequencies of the several component motions have values which are integral multiples of the lowest frequency present, the fundamental frequency. These multiples are two, three, four, five, etc. times that of the fundamental pitch. Thus even the most complex wave form can be analyzed as the interaction of pure, simple harmonic waves. The first clear association of tone quality with the presence of these component motions, however, was an empirical observation by Marin Mersenne in the first treatise on sound and music, *Harmonie Universelle* (1636).

> ... the struck string gives at least five different sounds simultaneously, of which the first is the natural sound of the string, serving as fundamental to the others ... I have no doubt that anyone can hear them who gives the necessary attention ...[5]

Thus the timbre of a musical sound is determined for the most part by the fundamental (first partial) plus what has come to be called the pattern of natural harmonic overtones or partials. The overtone series occurs in a predictable progression for any given frequency. For example, the second partial of C^2 (65 cps) is C^3 (131 cps), and the third partial is G^3 (196 cps). The first twelve partials for C^2 are shown in Fig. 29.

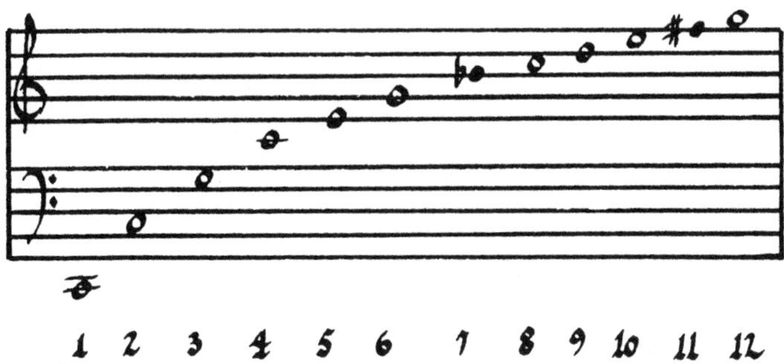

Fig. 29 Natural Harmonic Overtone Series

When an oscilloscope takes an electronic picture of a musical sound, the graph is like the one made by several tuning forks all vibrating at once, i.e., the sum of a number of simple pendular undulations with particular frequencies and amplitudes. Such a picture is called an "acoustic spectrum," and is the pattern for one complete cycle at that specific fundamental frequency and amplitude.

One often hears vocal quality described as "the number of overtones present in a voice." The matter really is not that

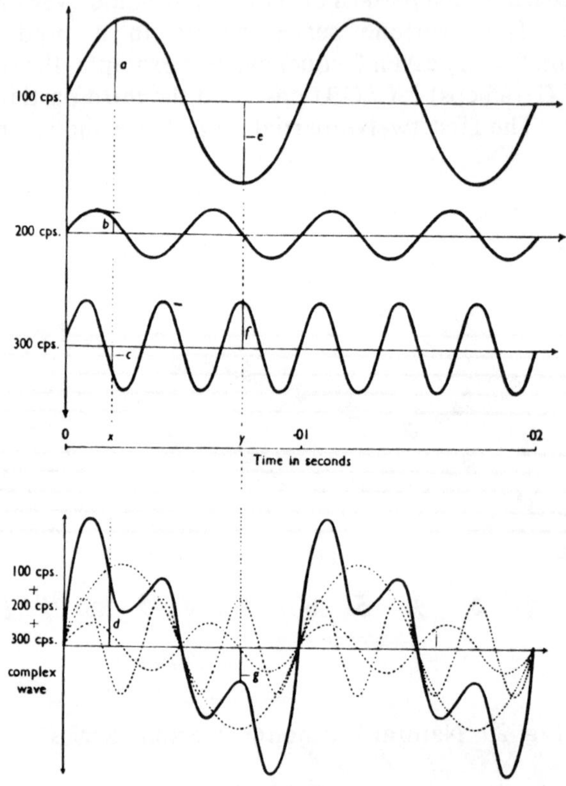

Fig. 30 Three Sound Waves Forming a Complex Wave (solid line represents complex wave generated by combining the three waves in A)

From *Elements of Acoustic Phonetics* by Peter Ladefoged, 1962, p. 35. Reprinted by permission of the University of Chicago Press.

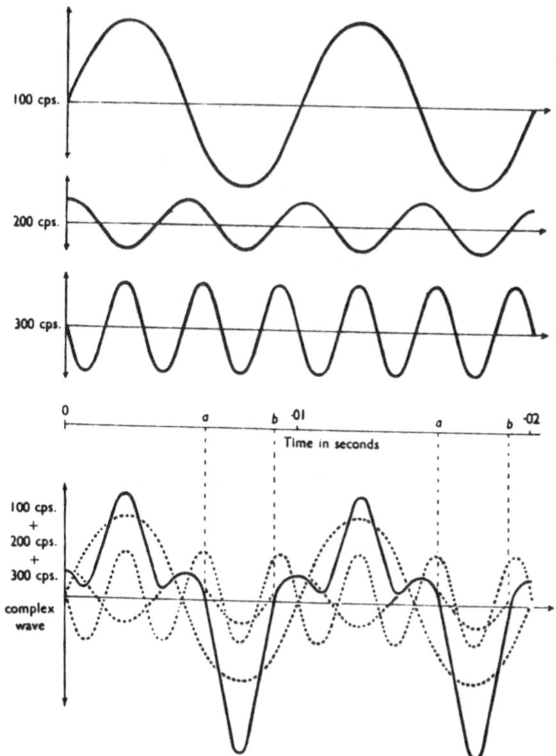

Fig. 31 Three Sound Waves Forming a Complex Wave (solid line represents complex wave generated by combining the three waves in A)

From *Elements of Acoustic Phonetics* by Peter Ladefoged, 1962, p. 40. Reprinted by permission of University of Chicago Press.

simple, and the statement is scientifically inaccurate. A complex sound wave consists of a fundamental or first partial and its natural harmonic components. The frequencies of these components and their relative amplitudes are important elements. Why then do tones with components having identical frequencies and amplitudes sound different from each other? Because their sound waves may have very different configurations, depending upon how each is increasing or declining in pressure. Notice the difference in the complex wave generated from the same three sine waves, but with different phases in Figs. 30 and 31. We saw the importance of phase at the beginning of the chapter and again in the section on amplitude. Imagine the significance of this element when many waves occupy the same resonator simultaneously. Resulting complex waveforms are strongly affected by this **relative phase** factor or differences in phase of its many sine waves. As Culver says, " ... circumstances may be such that two wave trains will arrive at certain points out of phase by a half period while at other points in the medium they may be only slightly out of phase. In such cases complete nullification will obtain at certain points and only partial or no interference at others."[6]

Whatever the complicated vibrational pattern of a complex tone, however, it is periodic and identical in frequency until the fundamental is changed. Since singing sounds are not simple sine waves like those of a tuning fork, future reference to a tone will mean a complex tone.

The sound spectrum reflects a specific timbre which is determined primarily by the following factors:

(1) number of partials
(2) distribution of partials
(3) relative intensity or strength of partials
(4) inharmonic partials (not part of the natural harmonic series)
(5) fundamental tone
(6) total intensity

In general, the more partials in the spectrum, the richer and more brilliant the sound. If one compares the tone of a flute, which contains few upper partials, with that of a violin, which is rich in upper partials, the importance of this factor is evident.

The distribution of the partials is also a strong determinant of quality. Each human voice has its own particular timbre, just as each person has a distinctive set of fingerprints.

The relative intensity of each partial also varies. For instance, two baritones may have relative similarity in the distribution of partials, but major differences in the intensities of the series.

If partials are present which are not exact mathematical multiples of the fundamental, they are called inharmonic partials and often tend to make the tone rough, unpleasant, or strident. Inharmonic partials generally have relatively high frequencies.

The location of the harmonic overtone series of a given fundamental also has a strong bearing on tone color. Low frequencies tend to sound darker than higher ones. Because the overtone series follows unbreakable natural laws, the tone color of a high soprano is of necessity different from that of a bass.

Finally, in most cases, the greater the intensity of a tone, the greater the number of partials present.

The Phenomenon of Resonance

Many musical vibrators, such as the vocal folds, a violin string, or the lips of a brass player, produce very faint sounds. They simply cannot be heard unless some means is available to augment them. Fortunately, the principle of resonance provides that help, and it is essential for singers and teachers of singing to understand this basic physical phenomenon. The quality and the focus of vocal sound are determined in large measure by how efficiently the resonance components of the instrument are used.

Galileo Galilei (1564-1642), the Italian astronomer and physicist, first stated the principle that every pendulum has its own natural period of vibration and cannot be induced to vibrate in any other period. Furthermore, the pendulum will swing or vibrate with wider and wider amplitude if the exciting impulses are properly timed. In other words, these impulses must have the same period as the natural period of the suspended body even while the amplitude increases. The motion of a swing is another example of the same phenomenon. You begin by giving a small push so that the swing moves away from you. When it moves back again and is at the top of its curve, you give it another push. On each occasion that the swing is given another push, it goes even higher. It increases its amplitude, the distance from its original rest position. If, however, you try to push the swing when it is still coming toward you, you slow it down. Only by waiting until the swing is about to move away is it possible to achieve an increase in amplitude. This kind of mechanical resonance occurs when the period of the driving force coincides with the natural period of the body involved.

How is resonance defined? It is the relationship that exists between two vibrating bodies and results in an increase in amplitude and a more efficient use of the sound wave. Optimum resonance occurs when these two bodies are timed to the same frequency. Wallis (1616-1703) made an early comment on sympathetic resonance.

> I have heard of a thin fine Venetian glass cracked with the strong and lasting sound of a trumpet or cornet near it, sounding a unison or consonant note to that of the glass. And I do not judge the thing very unlikely.[7]

No wonder every major operatic tenor in memory has laid claim to the same feat!

There are other common instances in which free sound waves activate resonating bodies. When one soundlessly presses down a particular key on the piano and depresses the sustaining pedal, each string becomes a resonator with a particular natural period of vibration. If that pitch (a complex sound wave) is sung near the piano, one or more of the strings will be set into sympathetic vibration, thus acting as resonators which mirror the spectrum of the sung note. The several frequencies heard correspond to the harmonic partials in the sung sound.

Vocal Resonance

The voice is a wind instrument. Air from the lungs is the actuator of the vocal folds, which become the primary vibrator and produce the sound wave. The air in the resonance cavity, the secondary vibrator, is set in motion in the period of the primary vibrator. The vibrator therefore imposes its frequency upon the resonator, unlike other wind and brass instruments. The resonating bell of the clarinet and the frequency of the reed are different. The bell determines the pitch and forces the reed to conform, and the player, understanding that the reed must conform to the pitch of the bell, may bite his reed accordingly. The trumpet player uses the valves on his instrument to make several sizes of resonating cavities, but he/she must vary the tension of the lips in order to get the full range of pitches. In the case of the voice, however, the resonating tract is tunable and can be altered enough to produce optimum resonance for the fundamental frequency and its associated harmonic partials. The more the resonance tract operates on the principle of sympathetic vibration, the better the vocal sound will be.

In the late 19th century, Hermann Helmholtz, the German physicist and acoustician, made a series of brass resonators. Each was shaped like a little turnip with a small opening at either end, one to be placed in the ear. For a sound to go through, it had to be timed to the same frequency as a particular resonator. When notes were played on the piano, the note whose frequency was close to that of the resonator produced strong vibrations in it, but the rest produced muffled sounds. The human body is not equipped with Helmholtz resonators, nor are our resonating cavities shaped as precisely and in as simple a form as his. Our resonators have an advantage over his, however; they are not made of metal. Metal resonators are sharply tuned and respond only to a few frequencies, whereas soft-walled resonators respond to many different frequencies and are able to reproduce many different gradations of tone color.

Acoustical Damping

If, by definition, sympathetic resonance adds volume and quality to the original sound wave produced by the vocal cords, then the acoustical phenomenon of damping is crucial to the singer. Damping is the time rate at which energy is dissipated in a vibrating body. It is the diminishing of the amplitude of an oscillation. In this case, the vibrating body is the air in the resonator. It certainly is possible that inefficient vocal fold action can generate a damping effect in the glottis during phonation. The resultant sound wave will then lack crucial partials or certain partials in the wave will not have sufficient amplitude to be adequately reinforced.

The degree of acoustical damping is dependent upon the vocal tract. As shown in Fig. 32, if the inner surface of a resonator is hard, the resonance peak is sharp, but if it is covered with an absorbent coating, the resonance curve is broader and less sharp. Transferring this concept to the vocal tract, the character of resonator walls, whether they are taut or soft, is therefore the first major factor. Generally when soft walls become tauter, the sound becomes brighter. Conversely, relaxing the walls produces a darker sound since the cavity is less responsive to the higher partials. Ladefoged calls this system an acoustic filter and defines it as a resonator "which is selective with respect to frequency; in other words, it transmits one frequency with greater efficiency than another."[8]

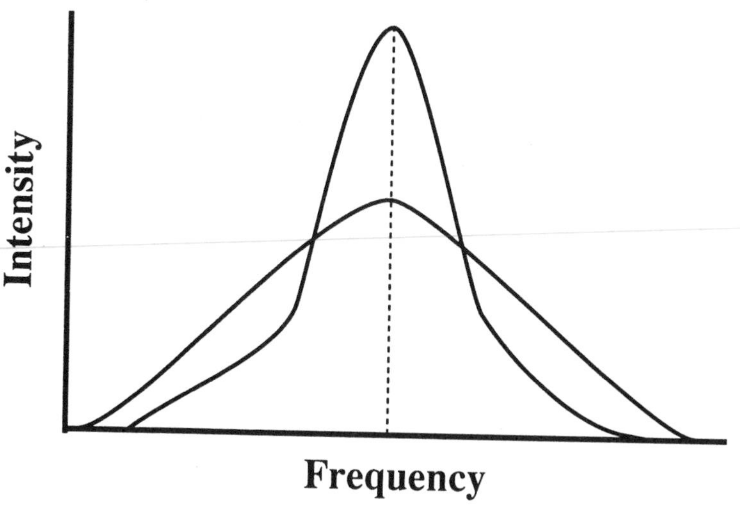

Fig. 32 Resonance Curves:
High curve sharply tuned with little damping.
Low curve a broader range with greater damping.

Secondly, if the size of a cavity is not appropriate for a specific frequency, intensity, and/or vowel, undesirable damping occurs. The conductivity or coupling of adjoining cavities is especially important for proper shaping of the tract. This topic will be explored in greater depth in Chapters 6 and 7.

The very nature of that fleshy cavity we call the vocal tract assures that all of our sound waves will be damped to a greater or lesser degree. The singer who knows how to appropriately minimize the damping factor, though, will be a gigantic step closer to optimum sound projection. He/she will get more sound with less effort.

If, on the other hand, the sound is heavily damped, amplitude is seriously reduced and vocal projection is poor. If a resonator is so heavily damped that the sound ceases the minute it is energized, we say that the sound is critically damped. When this kind of damping occurs, the vibrator zigs and the resonator zags; they work against each other, destroying the energy of the sound wave. The physicists says that they are "180° out of phase" (See Fig. 27).

It should be mentioned here that acousticians have differing theories about the factors affecting damped wave forms. The entire phenomenon, which is so essential to optimum resonance, needs a great deal of research.

Acoustical Laws Concerning Cavities

The vocal folds transmit energy in the form of sound waves and the vocal tract amplifies that energy. The resonator does not create energy, but it brings about the emission of energy at an increased rate. Since it acts as a filter on the sound wave, it has a major effect on tone color and focus. Thus operation of the force (vocal fold vibration) and the system (resonating cavities) according to the principle of sympathetic resonance produces optimum sound projection and the best quality for the singer. A "superposition" situation then exists.

Essential for an understanding of the resonance process are certain basic characteristics of the human voice. We now know that the waveform of a person's speaking voice is as individualistic as are his/her fingerprints. What is characteristic of all voices, though? What sets the singing voice apart from other musical instruments?

Olson[9] lists the following features of a vocal sound.

(1) The sound wave produced is a saw-tooth type containing the fundamental and its harmonic partials.

(2) The harmonic output (sound wave) of the vocal cords can be varied to some extent.

(3) The fundamental frequency of the wave can be varied at will over at least two octaves.

(4) Vocal cavities possess several different discrete or distinct resonant frequencies which can be varied, i.e., certain overtones can be accentuated.

Point four is the major characteristic which distinguishes the singing voice from other instruments. As indicated earlier, the greater the projection of sound, the more pertinent the focus must be so that a richer spectrum of overtones is present. Sometimes the resulting brilliance of tone is unwanted by the singer, who likes the inner feeling of a rich, round, velvety sound, but usually is producing a sound which is hollow, heavy, and lacking in projection.

One of the basic principles of physics is that every resonating body has a natural frequency of vibration which it will amplify to the greatest extent. The acoustical laws governing the resonance properties of a cavity are:

(1) **Volume.** The larger the cavity, the lower the frequency to which it resonates. The smaller the cavity, the higher the frequency. (Example: Blow across the tops of two bottles of different sizes).

(2) **Size of the aperture** (opening in an otherwise solid wall or surface). The longer and narrower the neck of the opening, the lower the frequency to which the cavity responds. The wider and flatter the neck, the higher the frequency. (Example: Blow across bottles of equal volume with varying neck structures).

(3) **Texture of the walls.** The softer the walls, the more the lower overtones are emphasized. Hard walls encourage higher partials. (Example: Sing in the shower; then sing in the living room).

(4) **Conductivity factor.** In the vocal resonance tract, coupling between resonators is achieved through use of the articulators, i.e., the tongue, the soft palate, and the jaw. (Example: Sing /**ae**/, then /**i**/, and observe the change in tongue position).

At the risk of stereotyping, many coloratura sopranos are small, not only in body size, but also in head size and neck length. At the top of their ranges, all mouth diameters increase, the walls of the cavity become taut, and a wide but short aperture is used. In contrast, basses and low baritones often have large and rather long necks. When they sound their lowest notes, their lips generally are pursed and projected (long, narrow aperture). Empirical observation of international singers in closeup on television amply demonstrates the acoustical principles of the wide cavity opening desirable for high frequencies and the correspondingly smaller opening for the lowest frequencies.

Variations in cavity volume and aperture configuration alone are not sufficient to account for the wide range of frequencies and colors in a singing voice. The balanced action of the extrinsic muscles has a major effect upon laryngeal positioning, which in turn helps determine the shape of the pharynx and the texture of its walls. In the next chapter, the role played by the soft palate, the tongue, and the jaw in shaping the resonance cavities will be discussed. This factor, the relationship between connected resonating areas, is called acoustical coupling, and is the mutual interaction of connected resonators as their joint air volumes are set into vibration. Adjustments of the articulators are used to change the length and diameter of the orifice or orifices between cavities. Appropriate coupling creates a wide variety of frequency and timbre possibilities in the human voice.

Although singers differ in the dimensions and the interrelationships of their resonating systems, the four factors listed above provide general guidelines which will be refined further in the chapter on vowel formants.

NOTES

1. See examples of this phenomenon in Donald E. Hall, *Musical Acoustics: An Introduction* (Belmont, CA: Wadsworth Publishing, 1980), 115-119.

2. Fritz Winckel, *Music, Sound and Sensation* (New York: Dover, 1967), 91-93 and 131-132.

3. Comparative figures quoted from Alexander Wood, *The Physics of Music*, 6th ed. (London: Methuen, 1962), 33-34.

4. Ingo Titze, "Male-Female Differences in the Larynx," *NATS Journal*, 44:2 (1988), 31.

5. Quoted in Wood, op. cit., 65.

6. Charles A. Culver, *Musical Acoustics*, 4th ed. (New York: McGraw-Hill, 1956), 38.

7. Quoted in Wood, op. cit., 26.

8. Peter Ladefoged, *Elements of Acoustic Phonetics* (Chicago: University of Chicago Press, 1962), 69.

9. Harry F. Olson, *Music, Physics and Engineering*, 2nd ed. (New York: Dover, 1967), 226.

Chapter 6

VOCAL RESONANCE

> The unique feature of the vocal apparatus is that the size and shape of the resonant system is under the conscious control of the speaker or singer.[1]

But is it? How many singers feel they can control the size and the shape of their resonators and if so, to what purpose? Do they know enough about the shaping of vowels to try to regulate their own vocal timbres, or do they sing by imitating their teachers' sounds? These are questions that merit serious and honest discussion wherever singing teachers gather together. Not all teachers have identical ideas about the nature of the act of singing, nor do they use the same teaching methods to convey these concepts. Differences in methodology are based upon aural perception and tonal preference, as well as upon individual personality, pacing, and previous technical training. There is certainly room for many kinds of pedagogical approaches so long as physiological and acoustical information about the singing voice forms the basis for the methodology. This instrument is irreplaceable.

Although certainly not a complete basis for teaching singing, a grasp of the basic physical laws of acoustics may prevent the teacher and the singer from striving for impossible or misguided goals and vocal procedures.

The Voice as a Wind Instrument

It is tempting to compare the voice to other instruments. Is it similar to an organ with only one pipe and a double reed? Perhaps in certain ways it is, but, unlike an organ, the vocal tract is made of living tissue and therefore can be altered in texture and shape. Can the vocal folds be likened to the behavior of stringed instruments? For both vibrators, three elements determine frequency--tension, thickness, and length. Both can produce rapid changes of pitch. The similarity ends there, however, because the vocal cords can change their tension while they are vibrating. Strings cannot. There is, of course, the more obvious difference between the use of breath pressure versus the use of a bow to activate the vibrator. Analogies with other instruments sometimes are useful, but beyond a certain point, they are inadequate.

It is generally agreed that the voice is a vocal-cord reed instrument, essentially a wind instrument of the double-reed type. The vocal vibrator is an air-stream sound generator which periodically releases and closes off the stream of air ascending from the lungs. The cords consist of two muscular wedges covered by membranes, each with one free border, rather than being a stiff lamina fixed at one end as is the ordinary reed. Not just the edges but the whole surface of these membranes is thrown into vibration. Considering the significant elements of the breath, the vibrating folds, and the resonating cavities, one can only conclude that the voice is truly a reed instrument.

The Resonance Cavities

There is universal agreement that the two principle resonating cavities are the throat or pharynx and the mouth, each of which is tunable; that is, their size and shape, as well as the dimensions of their orifices, can be varied by certain adjustments of the tongue, lips, soft palate, and jaw. These adjustments are under the voluntary control of the singer and must be practiced until they become automatic.

The pharynx is an irregularly shaped tube which extends from the back of the nose to the posterior surface of the base of the cricoid cartilage. Various sections of this large cavity are called the nasal pharynx, the oral pharynx, and the laryngeal pharynx. Arbitrary boundaries of these three sections are not intended as rigid dividing lines. What one person thinks of as the oral pharynx, another may consider part of the laryngeal pharynx. The entire space is a single functional unit and should be so treated.

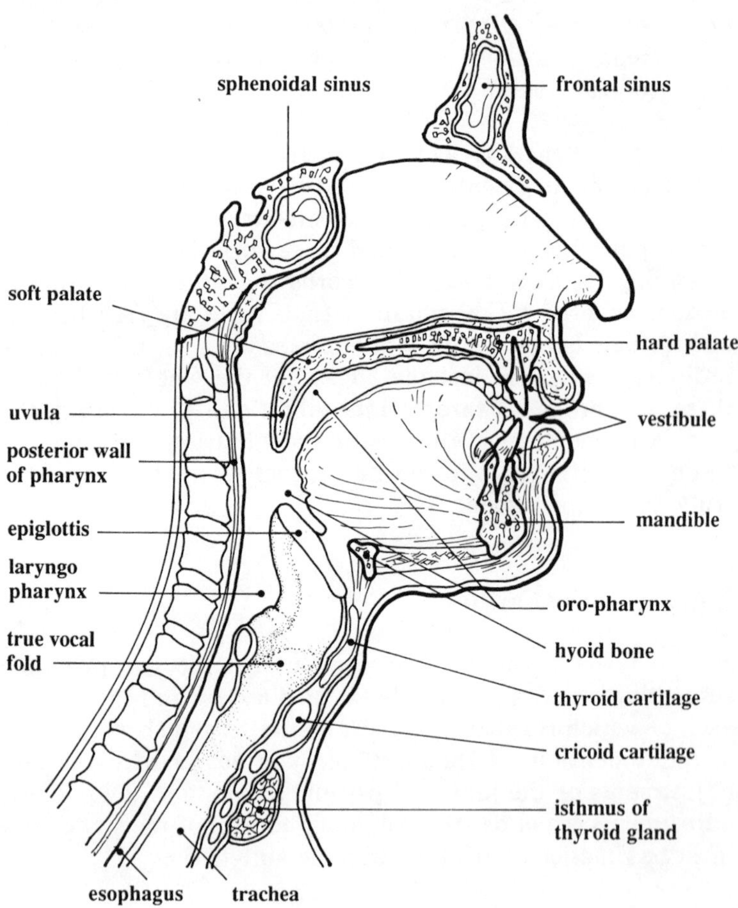

Fig. 33 Outline of the Resonators
and Related Organs

The nasal pharynx extends from the base of the skull to the soft palate. The palate acts as a valve and can close off this area, as it does in swallowing when food is prevented from entering the nose. The Eustachian tube, which leads to the middle and inner ear, has an opening into the nasal pharynx. In addition, there is possible vibratory feedback from the bones of the middle and inner ear and even from the cartilage of the outer ear canal. Because sound travels through bone much faster than through air, bone conductivity is undoubtedly one reason why the singer hears his/her sound so differently from a listener.

The oral pharynx extends from the soft palate to the top of the epiglottis. It is a large resonating space and has the greatest capacity for altering its shape, since both the soft palate and the larynx can move up, down, forward, and back. The position of the tongue also has a major effect on this space and its coupling with the mouth cavity.

The laryngeal pharynx extends from the top of the epiglottis to the base of the cricoid cartilage. Because sound waves pass through this area first, it is particularly important for the initial amplification of certain overtones.

Although opinions vary about the existence of possible auxiliary resonators, research evidence is discouraging, for the most part. The idea that "chest" resonance is generated in the chest cavity is a fallacy, since the thorax is not an empty cavity. It is possible that certain pharyngeal vibrations create the vibratory sensations felt or imagined by the singer, but there is as yet no factual evidence to indicate the use of the trachea or any other subglottic cavity as a resonator.

As for "head" or "nasal" resonance, many singers do feel vibrations in or near the maxillary sinuses directly under the eyes, and this sensation is as strong and as "real" as chest vibrations. Again, though, scientists point to sympathetic vibrations in bone and tissue produced by certain configurations of the vocal tract. The sinuses are not true resonance cavities, nor is the head, nor is the nose. Johan Sundberg, one of today's foremost acousticians, states the matter bluntly.

> Resonances outside the vocal tract (including the nose) do **not** contribute to the sound used in singing.[2]

Recent research, however, points to an actual auxiliary resonating space within the vocal tract. As early as 1949, Vennard kept an open attitude about the space formed directly above the vocal folds by the epiglottis and the aryepiglottic folds as an auxiliary resonator, a space which he called the laryngeal collar.[3] Subsequent investigation has confirmed that this little auxiliary resonator has a resonance frequency of 2500 to 3000 cps, and consequently generates the "singing formant," which is an essential ingredient of all good full-voiced singing sounds except those of high sopranos. Sundberg reports:

> It can be calculated that if the area of the outlet of the larynx into the pharynx is less than a sixth of the cross section of the pharynx, then the larynx is acoustically mismatched with the rest of the vocal tract; it has a resonance frequency of its own, largely independent of the remainder of the tract; ... I have estimated on the basis of X-ray pictures of a lowered larynx that this lowered-larynx resonance frequency should be between 2500 and 3000 hertz, ... just where the singing-formant peak appears.[4]

Sundberg attributes formation of this resonating collar at least partially to lowered laryngeal positioning. We have, therefore, another instance of functional interdependence in the vocal mechanism because if the strap or extrinsic muscles are not working, stabilization of the laryngeal position is not possible. The earlier section on interaction of the root of the tongue and its effect upon the position of the epiglottis also points up an important factor in the formation of this resonator. The fixed singing formant referred to by Sundberg is discussed in greater detail in the next chapter.

Tuning the Resonators

> In some cases resonators that are hopelessly out of tune may affect intonation; this explains how a singer with good ears but poor technic can sing "off key."[5]

This situation is little understood by non-singers, and even some teachers of singing and singing coaches continue to maintain that all singers with poor intonation have "bad ears." Maybe a few do, but the majority are experiencing technical problems. What causes resonators to be "hopelessly out of tune," and what can be done about it? Before considering the matter of vowel formants, let us investigate the articulators.

The Pharynx

Although the mouth and the pharynx combine to form a single complex resonator, the sound wave coming from the vocal folds must pass through the pharynx first. In 1894, Garcia said, "the real mouth of the singer ought to be considered the pharynx."[6] It is estimated that the first six partials are amplified primarily in the pharynx, and a great deal of the quality of the voice depends upon the shaping of that cavity.

If there is any single concept on which most singing teachers appear to agree, it is the idea of an "open throat" (not that they agree about how to get it or what 'open' means). The idea of an open throat apparently is a matter of interpretation and depends to a great extent upon differing aesthetic tastes in tone quality. For those methodologies which recommend a forward "placement," sensations in the nasal pharynx and oral pharynx mean that an open throat has been attained. For advocates of maximum space in the lower pharynx, an open throat has the opposite meaning.

Regardless of methodology, however, the pharynx should be free of constrictive tension, which causes bunched up, flabby walls and increases the danger of damping the sound. Because of its location, the lower pharynx is especially susceptible to distortion caused by a jutting neck. Unfortunately, pharyngeal constriction is particularly prevalent among English-speaking people. The back /ɑ/ is exactly that. The tongue retracts and protrudes into the pharynx, sometimes almost touching the back wall. What can be seen of the tongue through the mouth embouchure is not necessarily an accurate indication of tongue position, since the laryngeal pharynx and even most of the oral pharynx cannot be seen. A flat position is no guarantee that undesirable

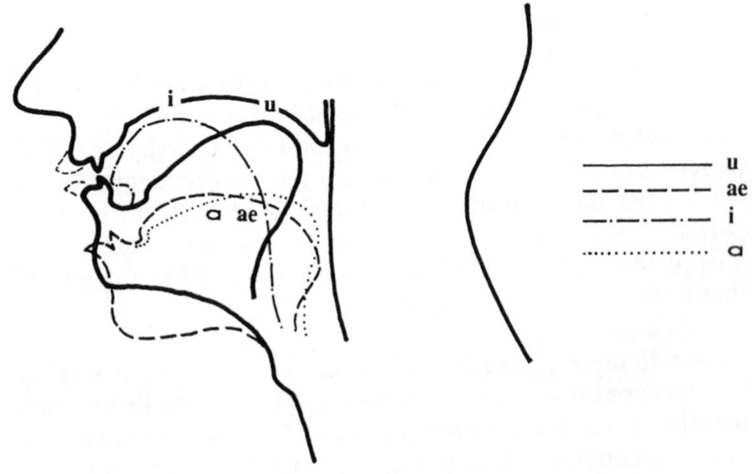

Fig. 34 Comparison of Tongue Positions for Four Common Vowels

tension and backing of the tongue is not present. The Italian /**a**/, of course, places the tongue in a more forward position.

Italian, French, and Spanish consonants are pronounced in a very different way from English and German ones. Most of them are dentalized, i.e., the tongue is fronted against the upper teeth and the air stream is not under as much pressure. The /**d**/ and /**t**/, for instance, are formed by a gentle movement of the tip of the tongue against the teeth. In contrast, the English equivalents are pronounced by bringing the teeth together sharply and releasing an explosion of air. The English /**l**/ is pronounced with the sides of the tongue against the molars instead of with the tip of the tongue against the teeth. Compare the Italian rolled /**r**/ with the infamous English growled /**r**/. The Italians and the Spanish form the /**g**/ and the /**k**/ with the front of the tongue rather than with the convulsive swallowing motion of the English. All of these undesirable and deeply ingrained habits of English-speaking singers can be changed by learning the responses which promote functional freedom. Singers should take the same phonetic care with their own language as they do with unfamiliar ones.

Another major cause of pharyngeal constriction is disuse of the extrinsic muscular network. If the depressors are not working in cooperation with the elevators, the larynx will ride too high, the root of the tongue will be depressed, and laryngeal constriction will follow.

The Tongue

The interaction of the articulatory muscles makes it difficult to isolate the behavior of a single muscle. It is probably correct to say, though, that the tongue is the most important single articulator because its configuration is the principal regulator of cavity coupling, for better or for worse. It occupies almost the entire vocal tract since it is fastened posteriorly to the hyoid bone, the epiglottis, and the soft palate. The front and the sides are free. Browne and Behnke called it "that big movable plug."[7] Effective resonation depends upon learning voluntary control of this large and often unruly muscle complex.

When at rest, the tip of the tongue should lie against the bottom teeth. Note that in this rest position and with the mouth completely closed, the tongue arches high against the hard and soft palates. This is its "normal" position, one which it assumes for more than half of a life span (unless you sleep two hours a night and talk most of the time). Intermediate positions between this normal position and the flat tongue have been learned for speech and for singing.

Movements of the tongue are greatly influenced by soft palate and hyoid bone action. The tongue can be extended, pulled back, raised, lowered, and made convex or concave, and any of these actions or a combination of them may be appropriate at a particular time.

> The quality of a vowel has its origin in the freedom of the space behind and above the tongue and in the freedom of the tongue itself.[8]

You will note that Shakespeare did not say the "size" of the space behind and above the tongue. Some vowels and some frequency levels require more or less space than others. Freedom and mobility are the key words here. Artificial manipulation of the tongue, whether by verbal directions or by physical means, is generally of no help whatever to a stiff, rebellious tongue. The more a singer is told to flatten the tongue, the stiffer it becomes. If the root of the tongue is being pushed and pulled about with a spatula, an oyster fork, or a miniature tripod, no self-respecting tongue will submit quietly.

Undue tension in the tongue often can be traced to tightness in the root. Self-extension exercises will encourage more mobility. With the lips and the lower jaw quiet and relaxed:

(1) Put out your tongue as far as it will go comfortably. Draw it back quickly so that the tip lies loosely against the lower front teeth.
(2) With the tip of the tongue against the lower front teeth, push forward gently. The tongue will roll forward and upward. Return to original position.
(3) Precede the vowels in vocalises with /θ/ (unvoiced /th/). It is difficult for the tongue to retract when it is continually asked to extend itself. Use of this consonant also loosens the back area of the tongue.

These kinds of exercises help the tongue to respond loosely and naturally. They are not spectacular, or even different. They do not get quick results, but they are effective and they do not substitute another problem for the one they are trying to solve. For the singer who retracts the tongue (particularly prevalent among Asian-speaking singers), these exercises are also very helpful, especially the third one. A retracted tongue forces the hyoid bone and the larynx into an excessively low position, resulting in a heavy, dark tone and muddy diction.

As a matter of semantics, it is best not to say "flatten the tongue." That phrase generally brings about a depressed back of the tongue. This kind of constriction affects the sound wave. Another direct interaction of resonance and phonation occurs, this time a negative one.

Few vowels are pronounced with a flat tongue. Proponents of certain singing methods still insist, though, that the tongue alone can form all the vowels, while the jaw is kept well open. It is suggested that each person make his/her own practical test and decide whether such a system is feasible. Even without empirical checking, however, it is self-evident that very little adjustment for vowel differentiation is possible. Typical of this method are continual instructions to "drop the jaw" and "make a bigger space in the throat." Because the upper partials are weakened under these conditions, the vowel becomes distorted, the tone is very dark, and intelligibility suffers. Richard Miller lists the following positions which often are the results of these singing methods.[9]

(1) The front of the tongue is below the roots of the lower teeth.

(2) The front of the tongue is curled upward and backward into the mouth cavity.

(3) The front of the tongue is against the lower teeth, but is humped forward over them in an exaggerated /**i**/ position.

(4) The front of the tongue is not in contact with the lower teeth, but is drawn directly back into the mouth cavity.

It seems only logical that the tongue cannot be in two places at once. It cannot be elevated and lowered at the same time, or fronted and backed, for that matter. Berton Coffin thinks the greatest variable in the throat is the movement of the tongue vis-à-vis the velo-pharyngeal axis.[10] His diagrams (see Fig. 35) and explanatory comments make the matter very clear. Vowels cannot have large spaces **both** in front of and behind the tongue hump at the same time. Either a vowel has

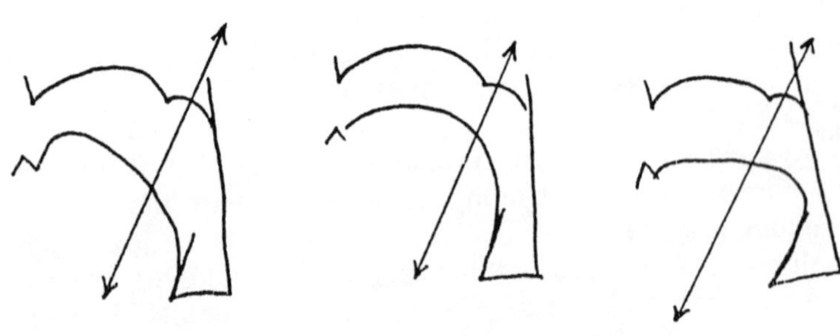

Fig. 35 The Velo-pharyngeal Axis

From *Overtones of Bel Canto* by Berton Coffin.
Reprinted by permission of Scarecrow Press, 1980.

a large space in the throat or it has a large space in front of the tongue hump.

The importance of the tongue is also noted by Howell, who calls it the primary articulator because of its role in cavity coupling.[11] Zemlin describes three general articulatory motions which shape the vocal tract.[12]

(1) The location of major constriction along the length of the vocal tract (where the tongue hump is)
(2) The degree of constriction (the space from the tongue to the roof of the mouth)
(3) The length of the vocal tract (determined by the position of the larynx and/or lip rounding)

The first two of the three are regulated by tongue position.

The best evidence of a free tongue is in the sound itself. Since the size and position of the tongue may vary from person to person, one cannot judge solely on observation. Some people have higher hard palates and the tongue can be more elevated without adversely affecting the sound. It depends upon individual size of the tongue, structure of the soft palate, and arch of the hard palate. For a well-balanced sound, the principal goal is to get the most favorable space for the needs of a particular vowel. This space, along with a relaxed tongue, produces optimum functional efficiency.

The Palate

The main purpose of the palatal area is as a separator of the esophagus from the nasal passages during swallowing. Its secondary function is as a resonance articulator. This area is comprised of the hard palate and the soft palate, and the height of the palatal vault has a direct relationship to the acoustic properties of the oral cavity and probably influences individual voice characteristics. The hard palate occupies over three-fourths of the total length, and the posterior one-fourth of this bony plate is formed by the palatine bone. For those few who still believe that the hard palate and/or the teeth serve as soundboards or reflectors of the soundwaves, that idea was refuted long ago. Hard palates would have to measure 20 square feet for low basses, and "a soprano might be able to manage with a palate of, say, six feet square, and teeth (if these are to be included) of the same length!"[13]

The other one-fourth of the palatal length functions as a muscular valve and is called the soft palate or velum. It consists of a complicated, interwoven system of muscles, which is directed posteriorly, and when at rest it hangs like a curtain into the oral pharynx. Since the soft palate can be raised, lowered, moved forward, moved backward, or tensed, let us look at the five primary muscles which are responsible for its mobility. There are two depressors, two elevators, and one elevator tensor.

1. *Palatal Depressors*

(1) **Glosso-palatine**. Runs from the front surface of the soft palate to insert in the sides of the tongue. Also called the anterior palatine arches or faucial pillars.

(2) **Pharyngo-palatine**. Runs from the soft palate downward to blend with the stylo-pharyngeal muscle and then into the side walls of the pharynx. Also called the posterior palatine arches or faucial pillars.

Contraction of the glosso-palatine will depress the soft palate or if the palate is fixed, it may raise the sides and back of the tongue. Since this muscle is semicircular, its action is sphincteric and will decrease the distance between the anterior pillars as well. The action of the pharyngo-palatine is more complex. We will only say here that contraction of the upper section of the muscle bundle is a swallowing and/or gagging action. When not so strong a contraction, a decrease in distance between the back pillars is produced. Too much upward or downward pull on either the front or back arches creates undue tension in an area where flexibility is of prime importance.

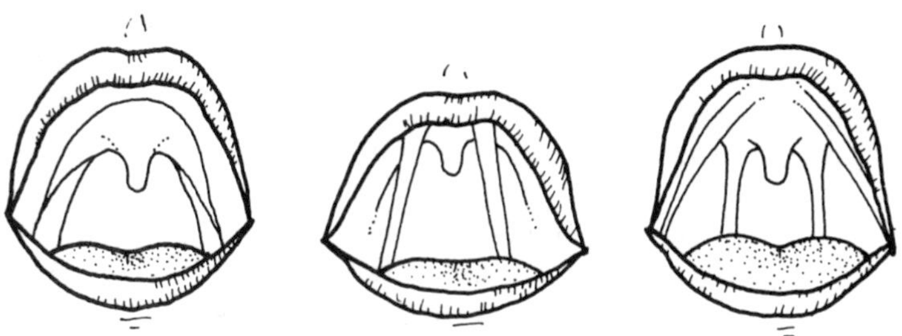

Fig. 36 The Palatine Arches

(left) Both sets in the proper arched postion
(middle) Glosso-palatine (the anterior arches) in a pulling-up position
(right) Pharyngo-palatine (the posterior arches) in a pulling down position

2. *Palatal elevators and tensors*

(1) **Levator palatine.** Forms the bulk of the soft palate. Arises from the temporal bone and the cartilaginous framework of the Eustachian tube and inserts in the palatine bone. Lifts the soft palate upward and backward and is important to velo-pharyngeal closure.
(2) **Tensor palatine.** Contracts laterally and flattens, tenses, and slightly lowers the soft palate.[14]
(3) **Uvular muscle.** Lifts the uvula, a midline pendulous structure, and with it the soft palate. Arises from the palatine bone, runs posteriorly the length of the soft palate, and inserts into the uvula.

It can be seen that, like the extrinsic suspensory network of the larynx, coordination of muscles which function as elevators and depressors is needed to maintain a free and mobile soft palate.

When a deep breath is taken, the larynx automatically falls and the soft palate rises, a physiological fact which has an important bearing upon change of tonal color and which will be explored further in the section on timbre.

In its relaxed state, the soft palate hangs downward, leaving the nasal port open, but in the elevated state, it creates more space in the pharynx and prevents an overly nasal quality. Vennard says that the velo-pharyngeal closure by means of the soft palate should be complete and that nasal resonance is of negligible value.[15] At the same time, he acknowledges the need for some "twang" in a tone, like salt in a cake, and believes that the use of "twang" in the upper range encourages "focus" and a strong singing formant.[16] Coffin shows X-rays of two famous singers, Amato and Caruso. While the nasal port is completely closed for Caruso, it is open in the Amato pictures except on the /**a**/ vowel.[17] What is especially interesting is that Caruso thought the velum should be open and was shocked that it was not.

As mentioned earlier, there is no evidence to indicate an auxiliary resonator outside the oral-pharyngeal vocal tract despite the presence of vibrations in or near the maxillary sinuses. There is still disagreement, however, about the velo-pharyngeal closure. Among singing teachers, some agree with Vennard's position, while others think that an excessively tight closure results in a harsh tone. Zemlin calls the fauces, that narrow opening created by the two sets of palatine arches, "the port through which the oral cavity communicates with the pharyngeal and nasal cavities..."[18] Studies by Fritzell indicate that there is considerable dimensional variation among singers, and as yet no conclusive evidence concerning what releases the closure.[19] The possibility of some kind of nasal-pharynx-mouth coupling while singing non-nasal vowels is being investigated.

Many singing teachers decry even a hint of nasality in the tone, but calmly accept and even advocate what they call "head resonance" or "nasal resonance". Is the difference between the two terms a purely semantic one? Is a fluid sound possible only when the arched palate feels buoyant and slightly forward? Does a soft palate held in a rigid, static position foster a vibratoless tone? Factual answers to these questions are not presently available. Until they are, any subjective definition of nasality and its semantic sisters must depend upon individual aural perception and timbre preference.

Jaw and Mouth Opening

Like the tongue, jaw position is not nearly so important as freedom of the hinge or mandibular joint. The hinge should feel loose and one should be able to feel a little space immediately in front of the ear. Particularly at high frequencies, the jaw must be very flexible and relaxed so the mouth can open sufficiently and the consonants can be pronounced very quickly with the tip of the tongue.

Although the subject is too specialized to treat in detail here, there has been an increased recognition in recent years of the prevalence of temporo-mandibular joint dysfunction (TMJ). In ordinary words, dysfunction of the jaw joint. Because the problem can imitate a wide range of physical problems and health disorders, it is frequently misdiagnosed. Symptoms often include nightly teeth grinding, pain in the jaw joint, a clicking sound when the jaw is opened or closed, dizziness, recurring migraine headaches and earaches, sinusitis, and soreness in the neck and back muscles. Oral surgeon Dr. Daniel L. Laskin, director of the TMJ and Facial Pain Center at the Medical College of Virginia estimates that stress-related muscular tension around the jaw joint can cause nine out of ten cases of TMJ dysfunction.[20] This tension produces muscle spasms or involuntary contractions that radiate pain outward to other parts of the body. It should be emphasized, though, that a clicking or popping jaw joint by itself is not necessarily an indication of TMJ disorder. Articles about the problem generally mention bite plates or splints, inlays or bridges, and other similar ways of restoring proper occlusion. Some do advocate biofeedback, but few mention facial massage. With an estimated 75 million Americans affected by TMJ dysfunction, at least 75% of them women, it seems logical to assume that stress in its early stages would respond favorably to a benign, kinesthetic approach like massage.

When the jaw is in its proper position, the head rests comfortably on the neck and shoulders. If the jaw is forced out of place, however, the muscles that support the head struggle to hold it in position. Severe muscular tension occurs. Sooner or later, the muscles go into spasm and cause little knots of pain that can lead to headaches, which is why TMJ is often diagnosed as a migraine.

Although it is true that emotional stress can cause teeth grinding and similar habits, particularly among persons who internalize their stress, there are also purely physical causes of TMJ. Burt Reynolds was hit in the jaw while making a film and suffered headaches and poor vision until his bite was corrected. Any kind of injury to the jaw, such as a whiplash from an automobile accident, or a birth injury, can result in a joint problem. The most common physical cause of TMJ dysfunction, though, may well be ill-advised orthodontal procedures, particularly removal of teeth for cosmetic reasons which causes the jaw to move out of alignment. The effect of TMJ syndrome on posture, on the extrinsic laryngeal musculature, and on the resonance articulators is devastating. For the singer it undermines any attempt to achieve functional equilibrium. Professional diagnosis and treatment are recommended.

Tightness in the jaw often is caused by other functional tensions. For instance, if breathing is clavicular, the extrinsic muscular network is deactivated. As a result, the larynx rides too high, the root of the tongue is tense, the jaw is tight, and pharyngeal space is constricted. Even the teeth and the large lip muscles may be trying to "help" by clenching.

The muscular network is out of balance and specific muscles are not working or are undertaking improper tasks. Conversely, jaw tension itself restricts or holds back air flow. It also constricts the walls of the resonators so that a pressed, shrill sound is produced.

Another common problem is excessive breath pressure or "support" on resonators which are not yet muscularly mature and therefore incapable of providing appropriate space. Such a condition is most often found in young singers.

Sometimes the jaw is loose before the onset of sound, but becomes set as soon as phonation starts. Such rigidity is characteristic of a glottal attack, or is often seen when a singer wants to "control" the sound.

The degree of mouth opening has always been a controversial subject. Garcia states that "the mouth should be opened by the natural fall of the jaw."[21] He goes on to say that "if this door were not sufficiently open, sounds could not issue freely." But just what does "sufficiently open" mean and what is the "natural fall of the jaw?" It depends upon the voice size, the pitch of the sung note, the vowel, the color desired, the dynamic level, and other factors peculiar to a given sound. Pavarotti thinks that "everyone will open and close the mouth as he feels."[22]

It should be noted, however, that the large mouth opening of the "dropped jaw" is not automatically a favorable position for all singing situations. Even a superficial understanding of acoustical laws makes this clear. Taylor's analogy, although funny and rather astringent, is justified.

> Many voice teachers encourage the students to open the mouth and throat as large as possible, apparently in the belief that if one tablespoonful of medicine is good for a sick person, then eight or ten ought to be that many times better.[23]

A review of the section on **Acoustical Laws Concerning Cavities** in the last chapter will re-affirm the place of cavity size and aperture configuration in the resonance picture. Mouth and jaw openings therefore are primarily dependent upon the frequency of the sung tone and the vowel used. Larger-than-necessary diameters not only are superfluous, but are detrimental. Adaptable, resilient mouth and jaw openings are functionally more efficient than fixed measurements.

The Lips

The position of the lips depends upon the vowel being sung. In general, the teeth show more for front vowels than back ones.[24] Vennard maintains that exposure of the edges of four upper teeth is "about right to give animation to preserve whatever good high partials have been generated in the tone."[25] Again, individual physical characteristics vary, and the shape depends upon what produces optimum resonance. Some singers use a puckered embouchure effectively, while for others the diameter of the aperture may be too narrow and result in excessive damping and an overly dark and muffled sound. The opposite extreme, a lateral position, can produce a metallic, even piercing sound if carried too far. The matter is subjective and depends to a large extent upon the shape of each mouth, the frequency of the sound, and the vowel being sung.

The lips and the large muscle encircling them must be relaxed and mobile. Their specific configuration is variable and has an effect upon the coupling of the oral-pharyngeal cavity.

The position of the cheeks also may have an effect upon the resonating space. Raising of the cheeks by both male and female singers in their high ranges seems to obtain maximum stretch of the soft palate without putting undue stress upon the palatine arches. This action can be seen in TV close-ups.

In summary, there is no one perfect position for tongue, soft palate, lips, or jaw. Each person's physique is different. The only unbreakable rule is that these articulators must shape the vocal tract so that the resonating space(s) can vibrate sympathetically with the sound waves coming from the vocal folds. Ideally these adjustments should be made with a minimum of effort and a maximum efficiency to avoid counterproductive tensions. The interdependence of the articulators of the resonance tract and the phonatory and breathing mechanisms is the key to attaining such maximum efficiency. "An inspection of the anatomical configuration of the vocal tract organs reveals that all the structures are networked by muscles and ligaments, suggesting that movements of the organs have an inter-dependency with each other. The tongue articulation, for example, may apply a force to the larynx, modifying its phonatory function."[26]

Timbre or Tone Quality

Timbre as determined by the fundamental plus the pattern of natural harmonics and their relative distribution and intensity was described in Chapter 5. Each instrument has a different characteristic tone quality, and for the voice, that most individualistic of all instruments, each voice has its own distinctive timbre or color. The basic color of each voice is influenced by the physiological features of that person, i.e., the body structure, the vocal fold size and configuration, and the supra-glottal resonance characteristics. After all the measurable factors are taken into account, however, one is still left with an aural perception which is extremely difficult to describe in words. Before grappling further with this generalized and subjective view of timbre, let us consider some of the specific ways in which timbre can be altered to reflect an endless variety of moods and emotions.

Four factors which determine the unique quality of each voice were listed in Chapter 5. The second factor states that the harmonic output of the vocal cords can be varied to some extent; that is, the vibratory pattern of the vocal folds is variable. As we know, the glottis opens and closes once during each vibratory cycle, and the number of cycles determines the frequency of the sound. The percentage of glottal closure time in a given cycle, however, determines the amplitude of vibration and the resulting character of the sound wave. The longer the closure time, the wider the amplitude and the stronger the upper partials. The interrelationship of subglottic air pressure and vocal fold resistance seems to be a major determinant of vocal fold amplitude.

> [A singer] can choose to have the cords swing with sufficient amplitude that they can press together during a controllable portion of each oscillatory cycle ... the flow consists of momentary puffs of air whose duration can be adjusted more or less independently of their repetition rate. As a result a singer is provided with an adjustable recipe for his internal sound source and therefore with one of his means for altering the tone color of his music.[27]

Shorter closure time and/or a less firm closure results in a narrower amplitude and a sound wave with weaker upper partials. Benade shows the two differing kinds of laryngeal airflow patterns in Fig. 37. The soundwaves in both graphs shown below have the same period or frequency. In the top graph, the flow rises quickly into a spiky peak, which after decreasing, ceases completely for about one-third of each cycle. This pattern indicates a greater number of high overtones and therefore greater intensity. In the lower graph, the wave form has a much smoother curve. A slow stream of air flows over the cords with just enough strength to keep them vibrating. The cords do not close completely, and consequently the flow is never shut off completely. This pattern demonstrates a tone which is lacking in overtones. The two kinds of sound produced by these laryngeal patterns Manuel Garcia calls "ringing" and "veiled," respectively.[28]

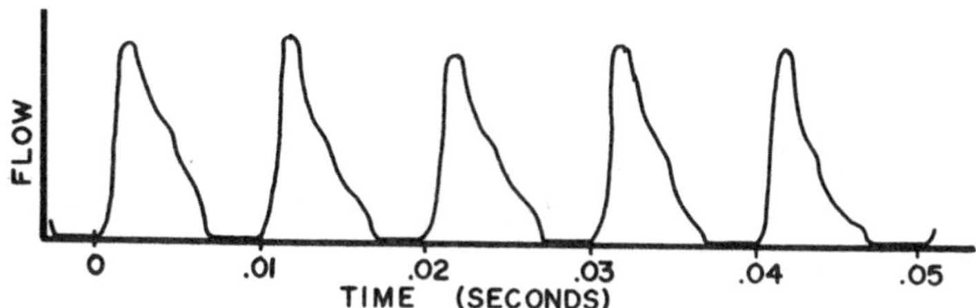

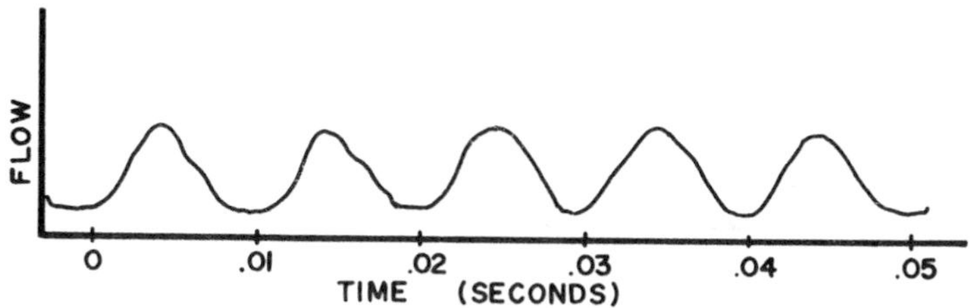

Fig. 37 Diagrams of Varying Airflow and Vibratory Patterns

From *Fundamentals of Musical Acoustics* by Arthur H. Benade, 1990, p. 368. Reprinted by permission of Dover Publications, Inc.

In more recent research, Colton and Casper maintain that "... the controlling mechanism of vocal intensity is not subglottal air pressure, (but) ... the degree and time of closure of the vocal folds themselves."[29] At higher frequencies, however, glottal resistance is no longer the major factor; airflow is. Although further research is certainly indicated, it is abundantly clear that the sound source (the vocal folds) and the supraglottal resonance tract have a strong effect upon each other.

In addition to the laryngeal method of changing vocal color, each singer can alter the form of the resonance tube. Brighter or darker resonance timbres are obtained primarily by the relationship between the soft palate and the larynx, which always move in opposing directions. When the larynx rises, the soft palate descends, and vice versa. Thus the high arch of the palate produces the darker timbre, and the lower arch the brighter one.

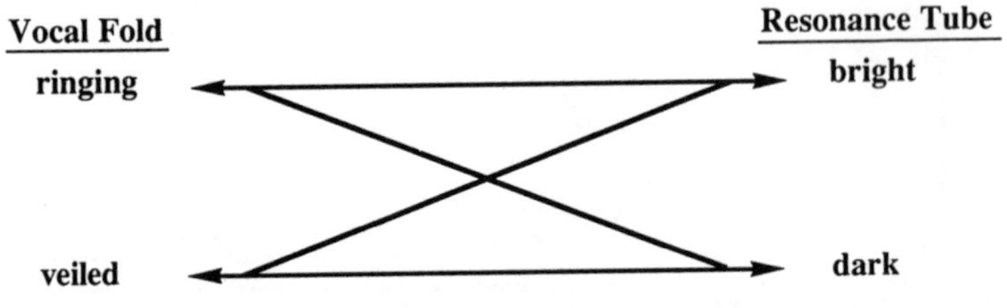

Fig. 38 Possible Combinations of Timbre

The singer therefore has at his/her command two major coloring devices. If they are used with discrimination, infinite gradations of color are possible. Garcia says that his observation about glottal closure, together with an understanding of resonance timbres and of the breath, puts the singer in possession of all the colors of the voice.[30]

Individual differences in articulatory behavior (and therefore of timbre) are the result not only of habitual "settings," but also of regional accents, language dialects, and personal ways of expressing emotion. Each singer's unique feeling for the words is revealed by inflection, dynamics, and the stress patterns that are employed.

Words have never been adequate for describing musical events, and they are even less satisfactory for describing tone quality. Such terms as "sweet," "abrasive," "bright," and "dark" all derive from senses other than the aural one and generally reflect personal preference or prejudice. Indeed, timbre seems to be a combination of physical characteristics, language differences, and aesthetic preferences.

Yet we have a tradition of using certain words to describe sound, what John F. Michel calls "an uncritical assumption of mutual terminology."[31] Until (and if) the physical determinants of timbre can be measured and labeled in the laboratory, verbal consensus is not possible. It is entirely possible that even then, individual psychological and emotional ingredients will preclude any standardization of terminology. In the meantime, ***chacun a son gout***!

NOTES

1. Culver, op. cit., 226-228.

2. Johan Sundberg, "The Source Spectrum in Professional Singing," *Folia Phoniatrica*, 25:3 (1973), 88.

3. Vennard, *Singing*, 1949 ed., op. cit., 51.

4. Johan Sundberg, "The Acoustics of the Singing Voice," *Scientific American*, 236:3 (March, 1977), 86-88.

5. Vennard, *Singing*, op. cit., 82.

6. Garcia, *Hints*, op. cit, 12.

7. Lennox Browne and Emil Behnke, *Voice, Song, and Speech* (London: Samson Low, Marston, Searle, and Rivington, 1887), 161.

8. William Shakespeare, *The Art of Singing* (Bryn Mawr, Pa.: Oliver Ditson, 1921), 32.

9. Richard Miller, "Supraglottal Considerations and Vocal Pedagogy," *Care of the Professional Voice*, Transcripts of the Ninth Symposium, Part II (New York: The Voice Foundation, 1980), 56.

10. Coffin, *Overtones*, op. cit., 13.

11. Peter Howell, "Auditory Feedback of the Voice in Singing," Chapter 11, *Musical Structure and Cognition*, Peter Howell, Ian Cross, and Robert West, eds. (New York: Academic Press, 1985), 259.

12. Zemlin, *Speech and Hearing*, 2nd ed. (Englewood Cliffs, NJ: Prentice-Hall, 1981), 354-355.

13. Richard Paget, *Human Speech* (London: Routledge and Kegan Paul, 1930), 211.

14. For further information about tensor palatine's complex anatomy, see Zemlin, *Speech and Hearing*, op. cit., 262-264.

15. Vennard, *Singing*, op. cit., 93.

16. William Vennard and Minoru Hirano, "Varieties of Voice Production," *NATS Bulletin*, 27:3 (1971), 30.

17. Coffin, *Overtones*, op. cit., 182-183.

18. Zemlin, *Speech and Hearing*, op. cit., 223.

19. Bjorn Fritzell, "Electromyography in the Study of the Velopharyngeal Function," *Folia Phoniatrica*, 31 (1979), 93-102.

20. Loryn E. Frey, "Temporomandibular Joint Dysfunction in Singers: A Survey," *NATS Journal*, 44:3 (1988), 15.

21. Garcia, *Hints*, op. cit., 12.

22. Luciano Pavarotti, Mizar Record PF3.

23. Taylor, op. cit., 31.

24. The terms "front" and "back" vowels refer to the position of the tongue hump and whether it is in front of or behind the velo-pharyngeal axis. Refer to Fig. 35.

25. Vennard, *Singing: The Mechanism*, op. cit., 119.

26. Kiyoshi Honda, "Variability Analysis of Laryngeal Muscle Activities," Chapter 10, *Vocal Fold Physiology: Biomechanics, Acoustics and Phonatory Control*, Ingo R. Titze and R. C. Scherer, eds. (Denver: Denver Center for the Performing Arts, 1983), 127.

27. Arthur H. Benade, *Fundamentals of Music Acoustics* (New York: Dover Publications, 1990), 363.

28. Garcia, *Hints*, op. cit., 7.

29. Raymond H. Colton and Janina K. Casper, *Understanding Voice Problems* (Baltimore: Williams and Wilkins, 1990), 291.

30. Garcia, *Hints*, op. cit., 7.

31. Lecture at Fourteenth Symposium: Care of the Professional Voice, Denver, Colorado, June 11, 1985.

Chapter 7

FIXED FORMANTS AND VOWEL MODIFICATION

What are formants?

A formant of the vocal resonating system may be broadly defined as a specific concentration of energy within the vocal sound wave. As indicated earlier, a vocal sound wave is composed of a series of simple harmonic waves with frequencies which are multiples of the fundamental frequency. What Johan Sundberg calls "this entire family of simultaneously sounding tones" is the sound wave that is sent into the resonance tract.

> The frequencies which are most successful in travelling through the vocal tract are called resonance or formant frequencies.[1]

Consequently certain partials in the sound wave leave the mouth opening with greater amplitude or intensity than others. The vocal tract resonances have given the vocal fold spectrum its final form.

These formant frequencies are shaped by adjustments of the lips and jaw opening, the tongue, the soft palate, and the larynx. Any change in the positions of one or more of these articulators produces corresponding changes of formant frequencies. The energized band of frequency and the resonating space are therefore identical. Resonating space = specific concentration of tonal energy or formant.

In the interests of reinforcing an understanding of what a formant is and does, we present another description of vocal tract adjustments and their effect upon the sound wave spectrum.[2]

> As the sound passes through the resonating cavities of the throat and mouth, the profile of the spectrum changes, since each cavity resonates to some of the tones in the spectrum more readily than to others and each adds its

> own characteristics to such tones. This reinforcement gives the partials greater energy at the point of cavity resonance. These points of greater energy are called formants.

Stated a third way, "a formant can be regarded as a peak in the frequency curve of the vocal tract filter. Thus, all partials are enhanced that are close to formants."[3]

Because all formants are harmonics of the fundamental, no formant can have a frequency lower than that of the fundamental.

An equally important point is that the pattern of partials making up a sound wave is determined by the vocal folds. No amount of resonance adjustment can reinforce a partial if that partial is not present in the tonal spectrum coming from the larynx.

The Fixed Formant Law

There are two basic ways in which formants relate to the fundamental frequency. In the relative pitch theory of tone quality, the strength of the partials is always relative to the fundamental. Stated another way, the strong partial(s) of a tone will always be in the same relationship to the fundamental. Thus the spectrum remains essentially the same provided the same register of the instrument is used. In the flute, for instance, the second partial is always the strongest, regardless of the fundamental. Most instruments operate according to this law of relative pitch formants.

The proportioning of harmonics in a singing sound, however, is almost entirely controlled by fixed formants. If a resonating space is shaped in a particular way, it has a given optimum frequency and will augment the partial(s) in the tone which matches its frequency. It is only a step further to the logical conclusion that if a vowel is formed in a particular way and a particular form has a specific frequency, vowels have pitch. The resonators are shaped by what vowel is being sung. This statement is not some unproven theory, but an acoustical fact which has been scientifically verified countless times. Every vowel, therefore, needs specific resonating spaces, and the shapes of these spaces have certain resonating frequencies.

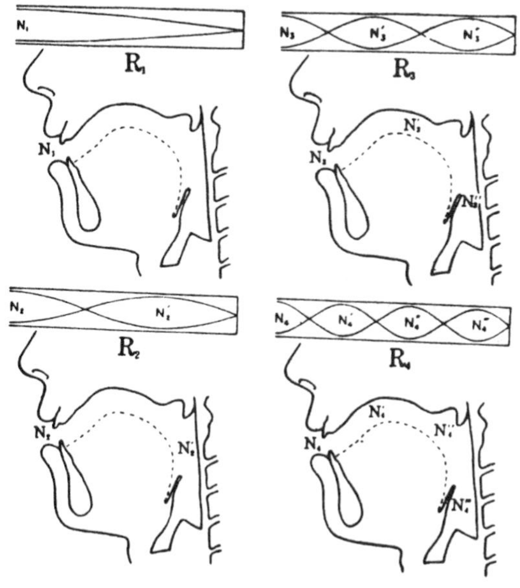

Fig. 39 Distribution of Maximum Points of the Volume Current in a Uniform Pipe or in a Uniform Vocal Cavity

From *The Vowel* by Tsutomu Chiba and Masato Kajiyama. 1958, Phonetic Society of Japan.

A singing sound, unlike the pure sine wave of a tuning fork, produces a complex sound spectrum. Sundberg believes that the complex sound spectrum moving through the vocal tract has at least five important resonances or formants below 4000 cps.[4] When a sound wave is fed into the tract, the closer a particular partial is to a formant frequency, the more its amplitude at the mouth opening is increased. These amplified partials manifest themselves as energy peaks in the spectrum, and certain patterns are characteristic of certain sounds. Each formant frequency is determined by the shape of the vocal tract. If that tract were a perfect cylinder (which it is not) and about seven inches long, which is indeed about average for the adult male, the first four formants would have natural resonances or formants at 500, 1500, 2500, and 3500 cps.[5]

Since the vocal tract is not a uniform tube, however, and its cross-sectional areas can vary greatly, these frequencies change according to varying patterns of articulation. Formants of women and children are higher then male formants for obvious reasons. For instance, there are some estimates that the average male pharynx is as much as 20% longer than the average female pharynx. Studies indicate that female formants are, on average, 15% higher than male formants, while children's formants vary widely between 25% and 40% higher.[6]

Since several simultaneous sound waves or modes of vibration are present in a specific air column, constricting or expanding the vocal tract in certain complex ways by moving the articulatory organs affects the formant frequencies of a given sound spectrum by either lowering or raising these frequencies. When the formant frequencies coincide with the harmonics of the sung frequency, however, the voice will benefit from sympathetic resonance and will gain in quality and projection. Maximum amplitude (super-position) is achieved.

Opinions still vary about how many formants there are in a tone. Recent studies confirm five major formants. The two lowest formants determine the vowel color, while f^3, f^4, and f^5 are "of greater significance to personal voice timbre."[7]

The first two formants are therefore generally called vowel formants and the higher ones quality formants. Let us consider the matter of vowel recognition by means of f^1 and f^2. As early as 1879, Alexander Graham Bell, inventor of the telephone, stated in the *American Journal of Otology* that all vowels are identified by double resonances. Along with Helmholtz, he laid the foundations of the acoustical law of fixed formants in vocal sound.

Bell used to give demonstrations of frequency resonances for the various vowels. For the first formant, he tapped a finger placed in front of the upper teeth. An easier method is suggested by Berton Coffin.[8] The changing frequencies of the first formant (f^1) may be heard by forming the primary vowels, /**i**/, /**e**/, /**a**/, /**o**/, and /**u**/ with the vocal cords closed. Thump with a finger on the base of the tongue below the jaw bone. The resulting pitch line is horseshoe-shaped ∩. Second formant frequencies (f^2) may be heard by whispering the same vowel series, resulting in a descending pitch line ╲. **Vowels have pitch**.

The energized frequency bands of specific vowels are at specific pitches. Despite variations in formant locations because of different vocal tract dimensions, the general locations of vowel formants are the **same** for both sexes. For instance, first formant frequencies for the /**i**/, /**y**/, and /**u**/ vowels have a range between 275 and 400 cps (approximately D^4 to A^4). For tenors and high baritones, this frequency is near the tops of their ranges, but it is in the lower part of the female range. These vowels generally are extremely difficult for women to produce an octave higher without modification. Approximate ranges for each vowel are relatively wide, reflecting differing circumstances and physical attributes.

The following chart shows frequency ranges for the two formants of commonly used English vowels. The traditional vowel triangle, based upon tongue positions for the various vowels, has been placed upon a grid, and the two formants necessary for vowel recognition are plotted.

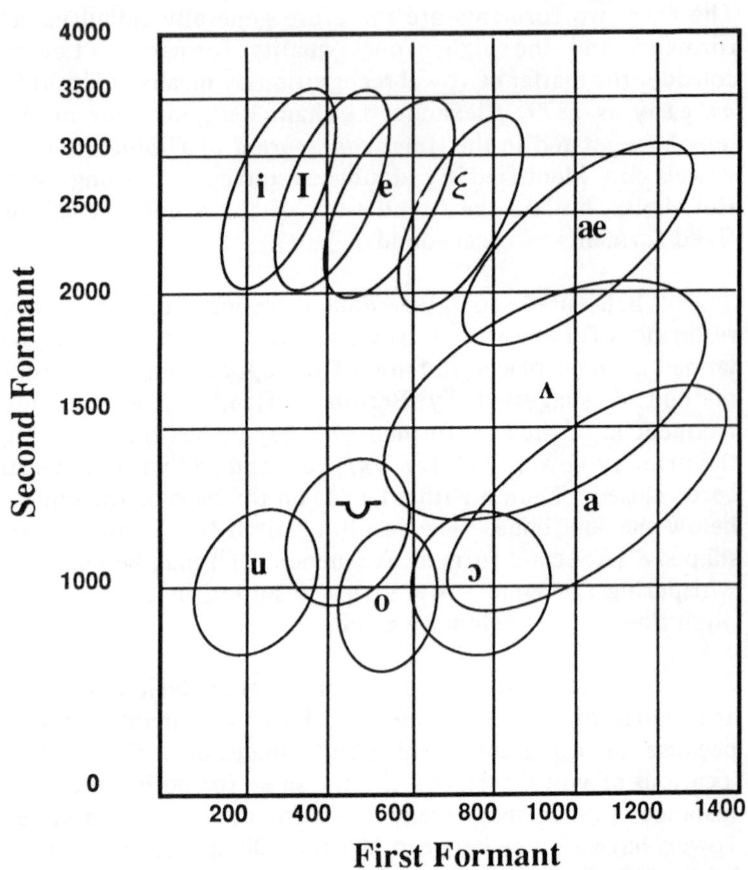

Fig. 40 Formant Ranges (based on data from Denes and Pinson, Luchsinger and Arnold, Wood, Vennard, Bunch, and Coffin)

It can be seen that there is some latitude for shifting formant frequencies before an original vowel color is so distorted that it is no longer recognizable. Benade finds that two people articulating the same sound will generally use slightly different formant frequencies.[9] Regional accents vary, and there are differences in the dimensions of their vocal tracts. Furthermore, no two people, irrespective of regional accents, pronounce a vowel the same way or even have the same conceptual understanding of how to alter the color of a vowel. Thus vowel formants will vary in exact location, depending upon a myriad of individual differences, not the least of which are variations in the physical dimensions of the resonating cavities. These differences are best treated through the discriminating ear of an experienced teacher familiar with the need for vowel modification. Whatever one's teaching method, however, vowel formants are an acoustical fact and must be observed if the singing voice is to be efficiently tuned and optimum sympathetic resonance achieved.

Vowel Formants and Harmonic Overtones

In the preceding chapter, there was a statement by William Vennard that resonators that are hopelessly out of tune may affect intonation. If we want to sing a particular vowel at a particular frequency, the resonators must reinforce a sound which:

(1) has partials of the fundamental (natural overtone or harmonic series)
(2) has partials within both vowel formants

If the second factor is not accomplished, the vowel will lose intelligibility and probably the basic quality of sound will be rough and the vibrato uneven. More importantly, if the first factor is unfulfilled, the tone will be weak and lacking in projection. Occasionally there will be no sound at all because a condition of critical damping exists. It is self-evident that the first task of a singer is to fulfill the requirements of the first factor and then to do everything possible to attain vowel fluidity and intelligibility.

The overtone series cannot be manipulated. Because its harmonic composition cannot be altered, the vowel formants must be altered to conform to the overtone series.

The vocal tract filter must act as a sieve which assists those partials whose frequencies are sufficiently close to a harmonic of a particular fundamental. Articulators must be kept flexible and mobile so that they can "hunt instinctively for the postition of best resonance at each change of the larynx note on any given vowel, or at each change of vowel on a given note."[10] A resonance tract with a set position is soon out of tune. Using the same size resonator for all vowels is defying natural laws.

A 1986 study by Darwin and Garner found that when a harmonic is mistuned more than 3%, it makes a progressively smaller contribution to the pitch of a tone. The harmonic begins to have fuzzy edges until at 8% it is completely excluded from the sound wave.[11] The researchers were investigating in particular the effects of first formant mistuning on pitch and quality. What a confirmation of Vennard's statement about resonators that are hopelessly out of tune affecting intonation!

What is sometimes called the instrumental resonance (overtone series) is essential for optimum sympathetic resonance, and vowel intelligibility must be sought through judicious vowel modification.

The Singing Formant

Before continuing with further discussion of the vowel formants, a more detailed review is needed of what appears to be a clustered fixed formant. This important formant lies in the neighborhood of 3000 cps, is completely **independent** of the fundamental frequency, and is known as the singing formant. It does not shift with a change of fundamental or with a change of vowel, but remains constant. Probably the reason it does not change frequency is because its resonator is independent of the remainder of the vocal tract. In the section on the resonance cavities, we described an auxiliary resonating space, a laryngeal collar directly above the vocal folds. If the diameter of the lower pharynx is about six times that of the laryngeal collar, the resonating frequency of that collar is isolated from articulatory movements of the rest of the vocal tract. An extra formant is amplified in that small space. Then, according to Sundberg, "the formants number three, four, and probably five are clustered and the ability of the vocal tract to transport sound in this frequency range is very much improved."[12] A 1989 videolaryngoscopic study using five professional singers found that "during soft, quiet phonation, the aryepiglottic orifice widens and the epiglottis is raised. When the voice intensity is increased, the aryepiglottic orifice narrows and the epiglottis lowers over the supraglottic opening."[13] This finding seems to imply that there is less energy in the singing formant when the aryepiglottic folds are relatively relaxed than when the orifice is narrowed.[14]

Another important factor in the formation of the laryngeal collar seems to be the lowering of the larynx enough to create stretching of the pharyngeal sidewall tissues and resultant widening of the lower pharynx. There is evidence that lowering of the larynx to a median position aids the clustering of the third, fourth, and fifth formants and produces the peak known as the singing formant.[15]

Of course, the singing formant cannot be amplified if it is not present in the glottal sound wave or if its amplitude is too weak. The amplitude of the high partials which make up this formant is highly dependent upon a fast rate of airflow and sufficient glottal resistance. The diagrams of airflow and glottal closure time in the previous chapter illustrate the nature of this relationship. When glottal resistance is high, the decibel level of the singing formant increases even more rapidly than the first vowel formant. In other words, lower partials do not get louder as fast as high partials when overall vocal intensity is increased. The singing formant, however, is not found in the falsetto voice, particularly the pure falsetto, and almost never in tones produced with a breathy, aspirate attack.

Sundberg says that the acoustical mismatch between the pharynx and the laryngeal collar cannot exist in the upper ranges of the female voice.[16] Bloothooft and Plomp concur and assert further that the singing formant is equally prominent in male and female voices until the fundamental frequency rises above approximately 400 cps, at which point the level of energy begins to decrease.[17] Above a C^5, presence of the singing formant is infrequent. Since the partials of higher frequencies are well above the strongest orchestral sounds, however, the risk of masking by an orchestra is slight. The high fixed formant peak in soprano voices is lower than for any other voice classification, and it is surmised that such a frequency is a normal clustering of f^3 and f^4.[18] Mean frequencies by voice classification are:[19]

bass	2200 cps
baritone	2700 cps
tenor	3200 cps
alto	2800 cps

The presence of the singing formant, signaling that ample high partials with sufficient intensity are present, is the single most important factor in a singer's ability to be heard in a large hall and over a full symphony orchestra. The full, "hooked-up" sound must be used. Rothenberg finds that under these conditions the sound wave contains the greatest amount of energy at high frequencies and will carry better above a musical accompaniment.[20] The orchestra has its highest level of sound around 500 cps, and the 3000 cps frequency of the singing formant carries the "ring" which makes the voice stand out. Actually, the singing formant is like a bonus to the singer. Sundberg says "because it is generated by resonance effects alone, it calls for no extra vocal effort; the singer achieves audibility without having to generate extra air pressure."[21]

We find that functional cooperation of the singing mechanism has become more and more complex, as well as more essential for optimum resonance. There must be efficient breath management to bring about firm glottal closure and the right kind of resistance to the subglottic pressure, and there must be proper laryngeal positioning via use of the extrinsic musculature.

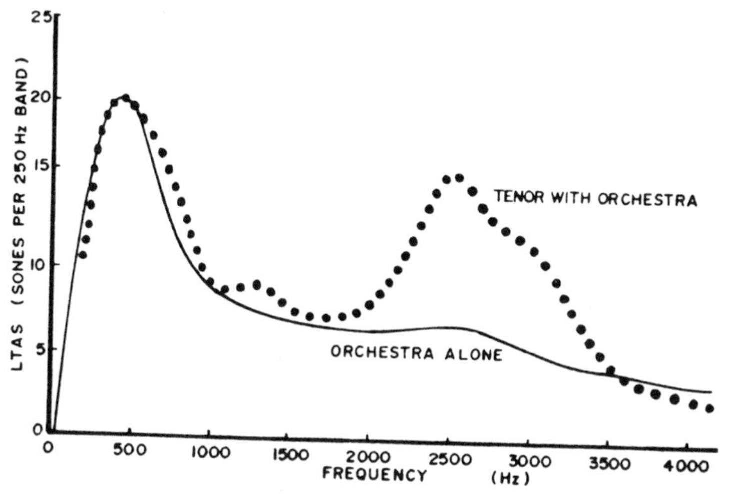

Fig. 41 Averaged spectra of the sound of a symphony orchestra without (solid line) and with (dotted line) a singer

From *Fundamentals of Musical Acoustics* by Arthur H. Benade, ©1990, p. 379. Reprinted by permission of Dover Publications, Inc.

With the singing formant playing such a crucial role in vocal projection, it is time to talk further about how to retain this advantage. Proper vowel modification will help the singer maintain good vocal quality and at the same time transmit the ideas and the moods of the words.

Vowel Modification

Tuning the Vowel Formants

Delattre maintains that there are two conditions which must be fulfilled to obtain good tone quality and vowel color. The first condition was covered in some detail in Chapter 6 in the section on timbre. The vocal folds must resist the breath stream strongly enough to produce a long glottal closure and consequently a richer tone. "Richer" means a larger number of

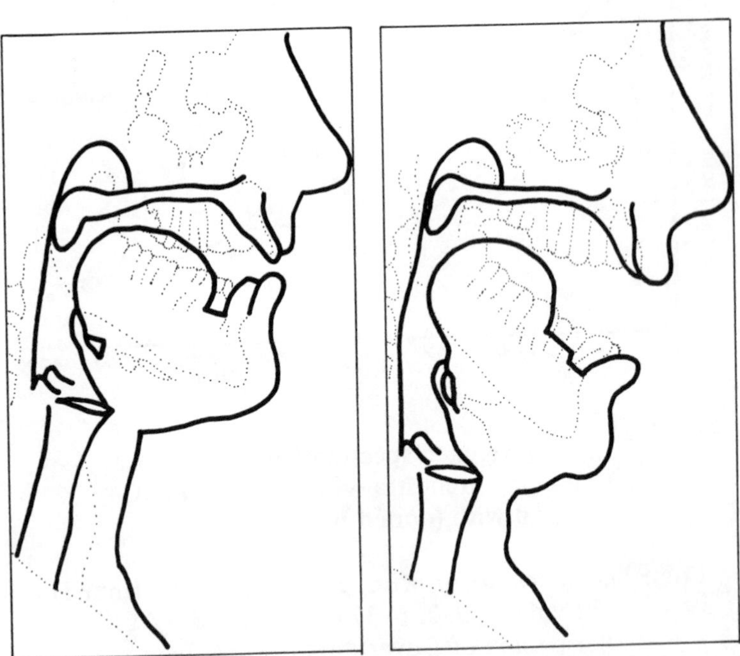

Fig. 42 Schematic of X-rays of the /**o**/ Vowel by a Speaker (left) and a Singer (right) at approximately C^5

After Delattre in *The NATS Bulletin* (October, 1958) Reproduced by permission overtones, reaching to higher frequencies, and with sufficient intensity. The second condition is that strictures or narrowing at the tongue and lips must be wider than for spoken vowels. "Otherwise, the high overtones that characterize singing voice quality cannot be 'passed' by the vocal tract."[22] Typical of efficient flow phonation is 60% open to 40% closed. Titze feels that the quality of the sound depends primarily on the "open quotient" so that the tone will not become "pressed."[23]

It is sometimes assumed that the first vowel formant originates in the pharynx and the second formant in the mouth. Such a view is oversimplified. These two cavities combine in complex ways, but never does the mouth resonate completely alone at one frequency and the pharynx at another.

Major tools for changing the shape of the resonating tube are the tongue and the jaw. For example, raising the jaw and at the same time raising and fronting the tongue produces a short and narrow front cavity and a broad and long back cavity. The cavities are loosely coupled because the influence of one section upon the other is not as great as if it were a single open tube. The above described configuration generates the lowest possible first formant (a large back space) and the highest possible second formant (a tiny front space). The vowel is /i/ (see Fig. 34 in Chapter 6).

If, on the other hand, both the jaw and the tongue are lowered, the two cavities are closer to the same size in a tightly coupled formation. The more open a vowel is, the less the mouth and pharynx act as separate resonators. Because the conductivity factor is very strong for the tightly coupled vowel /ʌ/, both the first formant and the second formant are determined by the overall coupling. It should be noted here that if the jaw is dropped too far or the tongue pulled down at its root, the general contour is seriously disturbed, and the epiglottis may be pulled forward unduly as well. This kind of tension also constricts the lower pharyngeal walls.

There are two major articulation factors which are critical in formant shaping.

(1) Location of the area of maximum constriction (the orifice), accomplished by backing or fronting the tongue
(2) Size of this area of constriction, accomplished by raising or lowering the tongue to and from the roof of the mouth

For front vowels, f^1 rises as the tongue lowers and the cross-sectional area of the internal orifice increases (factor two above), as in, for example, the progression of /**i**/, /**I**/, /**e**/, and /ɛ/. Conversely, this same action decreases the f^2 frequency.

For back vowels, the constriction in the oral pharynx during the /ɑ/, /ɔ/, /ʊ/, /**u**/ series moves forward (factor one above) and f^1 decreases as the back space becomes larger. It is intriguing to note that some researchers find that the location of the orifice for /**u**/ is not significantly farther back than for /**i**/. The same study finds that /**æ**/ and /**o**/ can be more convincingly paired on the basis of tongue behavior than can /**æ**/ and /**a**/.[24] These two statements have fascinating articulatory implications for singers.

For all back vowels, a third articulatory factor enters the picture. "All formant frequencies decrease uniformly with lip rounding and increase with lip spreading,"[25] thus explaining some of the difference in ring and intensity between /**u**/ and /**i**/. It should be mentioned also that for many of these back vowels, a slightly wider mouth opening than that used in speech will raise and strengthen the formants. Fant agrees that lip rounding lowers all resonance frequencies.[26] Try rounding the lips over an /**a**/ vowel to produce an /ɔ/.

It is interesting to note that pursing of the lips for umlauts, which are puckered front vowels (the tongue is fronted) does not affect f^1 much, but the higher formants are lowered considerably. For instance, the fourth formant, which generally is higher than the singing formant (f^5) for /œ/, /**ø**/, /**y**/, and /**Y**/, is lowered, and the intensity of the singing formant is enhanced by this clustering action.[27]

The articulation of formant patterns must be thought of in correlational terms, not as single factors. The two cavity volumes can seldom be varied independently. In general, for front vowels, a lowering of the tongue causes an increase in conductivity between the cavities and a front volume increase. Consequently, f^2 decreases and f^1 increases (as it does from /**e**/ to /ɛ/, for instance). If the tongue rises and fronts, f^2 increases and f^1 decreases (as it does when going from /ɛ/ to /**e**/).

For back vowels, the oral cavity changes volume less than does the back cavity, primarily because tongue raising and lowering is not as great. Formant patterns are influenced more by total length and the degree of lip rounding. For instance, the first formant of /**u**/ is tuned much more by lip formation than by tongue constriction. For back vowels, then, coupled cavity volume and total length effect both formants. Titze says that "all formant frequencies decrease uniformly as the length of the vocal tract increases."[28] Apparently the increase or decrease is about 10%, but such a seemingly small percentage will have a measurable effect on vowel color. To the common articulators of jaw, tongue, and lips, then, we must add:

(1) the position of the larynx, which determines the vocal tract length
(2) the position of the walls of the pharynx, determined primarily by soft palate configuration

Sundberg thinks that these two factors affect all formant frequencies, including f^3, f^4, and f^5, and their degree of clustering.[29]

Resonance tract configurations for specific vowels are noted below.

(1) Tongue is backed for /**u**/ and /**o**/, but higher for /**u**/ than /**o**/. The /**a**/ is more fronted than /**o**/, and lower.

(2) Tongue is fronted for /**i**/ and /**e**/, but higher for /**i**/ than /**e**/. The /**I**/ vowel occupies a position between them.

(3) /**æ**/, a very open front vowel, has a maximum front resonating space and a very small back space. The wide formant range for this vowel shown in Fig. 40 probably reflects variations in the degree of cross-sectional stricture in the back cavity.

(4) For /**a**/ and lateral /˘/, f^1 and f^2 are relatively close (approximately 780 and 1240). A simultaneous slight shifting of frequencies to increase f^1 and decrease f^2 will allow the two frequencies to merge into a single band with a much higher intensity level.

Nasalization is difficult to characterize because it varies widely both with the singer and with the type of nasal coupling being used, i.e., whether a pure murmur, a nasalized vowel, such as the French ones, or some intermediate sound. Within the nasal murmur, all high formant levels are greatly reduced in frequency and amplitude. Fant reports that the f^2 of /**m**/ is higher than that of /**n**/.[30] The most widely agreed upon finding about nasalized vowels is that the first formant is greatly reduced in intensity. Furthermore, Fant and other researchers (Delattre [1954] and House and Stevens [1956]) noted in oscillograms that vowels preceded by nasal consonants are much more heavily damped than those preceded by other consonants.[31] The implications for singing in large halls and with orchestras are obvious.

The first two formants have a vital effect upon vowel color and intelligibility. They also have a major effect upon overall tone quality. In fact, there is increasing evidence that vowel quality and musical timbre are similar facets of a common acoustical base. Even small changes in the two vowel formants make large differences in timbre. By tuning these formants of the resonating tube, better quality and greater intensity can be achieved with less effort. Sundberg estimates that a singer can get as much as a 30 dB increase in sound level by means of resonance tuning alone![32]

The Importance of the First Formant

The importance of first formant tuning cannot be over-emphasized, as it always contributes more to the total intensity than any other formant. Although f^1 tuning generally depends upon the entire vocal tract, the frequency range of the pharynx defines the upper limits of f^1 frequencies to some extent. To be sure, these upper limits can be raised by certain kinds of cavity coupling and perhaps even by other kinds of pharyngeal manipulation not yet identified. Why some high female voices successfully negotiate pitches above F^5 with less vowel modification than others is not well understood ("Not well understood" is a scientist's way of saying that little research has been done on the specific subject, and what has been done produced unclear implications). From an empirical standpoint, small, bright voices with high tessituras generally need less cavity adjustment by means of vowel modification than bigger, darker voices.

Coffin estimates an average frequency range of 350 to 750 cps for the pharyngeal cavity,[33] and Sundberg cites 250 to 700 cps for adult males.[34] The real importance of these figures is that the first formants of all vowels except open tube ones (/**a**/, /æ/, and /ʌ/) lie in this frequency range of D^4 at 293 cps to F^5 at 698 cps. For all frequencies above D^4, which means the high ranges of baritones and tenors plus all female ranges except the lowest alto notes, the singer must learn how to alter his/her vocal tract to match the appropriate vowel formant frequency with the fundamental being sung. See the next section on matching formants and the harmonic series for further investigation of the pharynx and first formants. A table by Coffin, shown below, lists average f^1 frequencies. Similar charts by Peterson and Barney (1952) and Howie and Delattre (1962) show somewhat lower figures, presumably because of the difference in male and female formants.

æ	a	ɑ	750 cps	(F♯^{5})
ɛ	œ	ɔ	600 cps	(D^5)
e	ø	o	456 cps	(A^4)
i	y	u	350 cps	(F^4)

Fig. 43 First Formant Frequencies (after Coffin)

Matching Formants and the Harmonic Series

Singers must be able to match their f^1 vowel frequencies to the harmonic or instrumental resonance of the sung pitch or else a weakening and distuning of vocal cord vibration will result:

> There is good evidence that when we are learning the shape of the cavities above the larynx, we are training the vocal cords unconsciously at the same time.[35]

Although that concept was initially stated in 1949 when the first edition of Vennard's book was published, it is no longer a new or startling hypothesis. Its validity is affirmed by voice scientists and acousticians throughout the world. Appropriate shaping of the supraglottal resonance tract increases the amplitude of the vibrating vocal folds while also lessening the adductive or muscular force needed by the folds. Rothenberg (1988) suggests that those frequencies near register bridges or other areas in which the oscillatory mechanism is being stretched to its limit are especially affected by the acoustical properties of the resonance tract. " ...singers may be expected to vary in the degree to which they employ tuning to create pressure-flow phase relationships at the glottis that maximize the oscillatory energy in the vocal folds ..."[36] The same concept is expressed by Coffin.

> ... air pressures move from the source to the mouth of the instrument and a portion of the pressures is reflected back upon the vibrating sound source assisting it in its vibration.[37]

A 1982 article by Ingo Titze puts forth the same principle.[38]

> "Different vowels, for example, create different degrees of loading on the vocal folds. We have all experienced this, but it has now been demonstrated scientifically that ***not only can vowel modification optimize the resonance for a given source, but the source itself can be strengthened by tuning for optimal loading conditions.***" (emphasis added)

Simply stated, vowel modification can produce changes in glottal airflow and pressure, which in turn alter the vibratory pattern of the vocal folds. Because the concept is so little understood by vocal pedagogs, yet so central to efficient functioning of the singing voice, we quote from a 1992 study using five professional tenors and 25 control subjects. While investigating how the vocal tract affects the power produced at the glottis, the researchers found that an appropriate vocal tract configuration provided a 10-15 decibel increase in sound pressure level. At higher fundamental frequencies, an additional 3-5 decibels are possible when the vowel formants are finely tuned to the harmonics of the sound wave. "... singers learn how to lower their effective glottal impedance to transfer more power from the source to the vocal tract for a given lung pressure."[39] Acoustic output power is boosted when the frequency of a formant coincides with the frequency of a harmonic.

In addition to a more efficient and less forceful use of the vocal folds, resonance tuning can minimize air consumption, especially at high frequencies. When the first formant is close to the fundamental frequency, air expenditure is reduced markedly.[40]

Even though formants are bands of frequency and subject to the individual differences discussed earlier, the average first formant frequencies are charted below for purposes of illustration. The chart also will help readers become familiar with the approximate locations of f^1 frequencies.

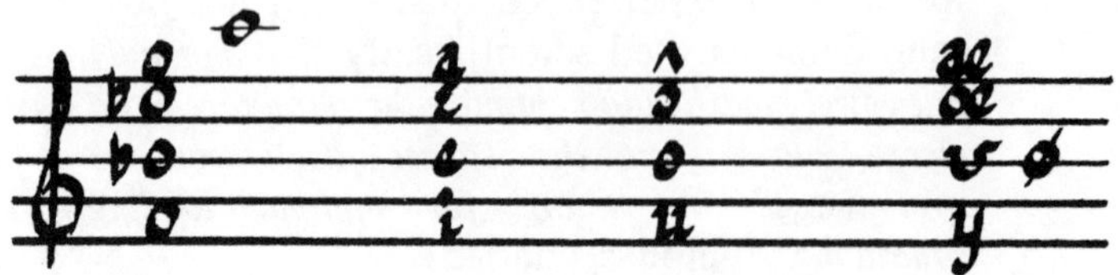

Fig. 44 Mean Frequencies of First Formants

An example of how vowel shading can achieve optimum first formant tuning is shown in the illustration below. In the chart at the left, a baritone or tenor is singing the /ε/ vowel on C^3, while the right chart shows a mezzo soprano singing the same vowel on G^3. The mezzo sound spectrum shows a high concentration of energy on the third partial, D^5, in the approximate location of the first formant of the /ε/ vowel. For the male singer, energy peaks on either the fourth partial (first formant of /**e**/) or the fifth partial (first

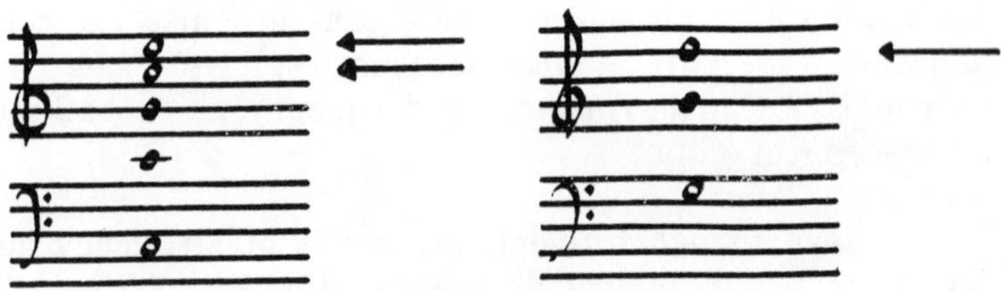

Fig. 45 Baritone or Tenor (left) and Mezzo (right) singing the /ε/ vowel. Arrows show locations of energy peaks (formants)

formant of /ε/). Either are possible, depending upon such variables as size of voice, classification, anatomical features, and dynamic level. Sympathetic resonance and better tone quality depend upon approximate vowel shading.

Above approximately 270–350 cps, the singer must match the vowel formant to the fundamental of the tone. Men obtain sympathetic resonance by seeking a match between vowel formants and the harmonic series, except for their high ranges (pitches above approximately D^4). Women rely primarily upon vowel modifications for reinforcement at the fundamental. Again, men and women should NOT be trained alike so far as vowel modification is concerned.

For a fundamental pitch higher than the f^1 frequency of a particular vowel, the formant must be raised to conform to the fundamental or first partial. For instance, a soprano or mezzo is required to sing the /**u**/ vowel on $B\flat^4$ (494 cps), which clearly lies above the first formant of /**u**/ (approximately 350 cps). She therefore alters her tongue, jaw, and lip positions slightly in order to raise this first formant to match the fundamental frequency she is singing. The most likely choice for her is the /ʊ/ at about 400 cps, or even a slight modifying toward /**o**/, which is in the same general frequency area. Experimentation and careful listening will determine which is right for a specific singer. Too severe a migration to a vowel like /ɔ/ at about 600 cps will be counter-productive, and neither instrumental resonance nor vowel intelligibility will be served.

When f^1 is matched to the instrumental resonance, there is a minimal variation of dynamics from pitch to pitch and from vowel to vowel, and the vibrato is even and fluid. The happy result is that most sought after of vocal goals, a legato line. To the singer's joy, there is even a bonus:

> ... the most obvious advantage that comes from even an approximate tuning of the first formant is a very large increase in the loudness

> of the sound a singer can achieve for a given vocal effort.[41]

Benade goes on to say that not only is such a result essential for singing in large halls and with orchestras, but it also increases the singer's dynamic range. In other words, even a pianissimo has body and projection if it is sung with sympathetic resonance.

Operatic composers writing before the age of acoustical research may not have known the scientific principle of fixed vowel formants, but they certainly listened to singers and used the empirical knowledge gained. Pagliacci sings "ridi, Pagliacci" with the /i/ vowel's high, intense second formant plus the first formant frequency matching the fundamental frequency he is singing (G^4 and $F\sharp^4$). No wonder that despairing cry has thrilled opera audiences for decades! Look at other famous tenor arias, and you will find numerous high A's and B♭'s on the /e/ vowel. Tenors love these vowels, but must be careful to get enough "rumble" or back cavity resonance to balance those ringing overtones. Most /i/ vowels in the male passaggio need a little /y/ to provide more pharyngeal space and to lower the higher formants to produce the clustering needed for the singing formant. Then the Italian concept of ***chiaroscuro*** is well served, and the sound has what is commonly called "cover." Covered singing is characterized by a comfortably low laryngeal position, a strong fundamental, appropriate vowel modification and a rich spectrum of higher harmonics. Once again the functional unity of fluid breathing, use of the extrinsic muscles for laryngeal positioning, and optimum resonance tuning is the key.

The First Vowel Formant and the Soprano Voice

Sundberg believes that the higher a soprano sings, the wider her jaw is opened so that the first formant frequency can be matched to the frequency of the sung tone.[42]

To state this acoustical law once again, if the fundamental frequency of the sung note is higher than the first formant of the vowel being sung, the fundamental frequency itself must serve as the first formant and the vowel color altered to match that frequency. A 1977 study of the soprano voice shows that achieving an even scale is not solely a matter of skillfull handling of breath and phonatory cooperation, but also of articulation, i.e., formant shifts. Advantages gained by the soprano or mezzo-soprano who matches f^1 to fundamental frequency at the higher pitches are:[43]

(1) "strong sounds at the lowest possible price in vocal effort"
(2) avoidance of variations in quality on successive pitches and particularly at register bridges (especially desirable at chest-middle voice bridge)
(3) avoidance of substantial unintentional loudness variations on successive pitches
(4) less loss of intelligibility regardless of pitch, compared with singing the "pure" vowel

It seems probable, then, that in addition to breath management and vocal fold factors, first formant tuning is a crucial factor in achieving smooth register transitions as well as maintaining as much vowel integrity as possible.

Only /**a**/, /ɑ/, /æ/, and /ʌ/ have first formant frequencies above F^5. Since these are laboratory figures, we find that some sopranos can produce close approximations of other vowel sounds in the upper passaggio. Perhaps the resonators reinforce auxiliary formants that affect the quality. In the higher ranges, however, the problem must be solved by other means, since the mouth cavity tends to run short of partials and the pitch is far above the range of the pharyngeal cavity. A satisfactory /**u**/ or /**i**/ above F^5 is rare without at least some vowel modification. The higher the soprano sings, the more instrumental her tone becomes as the resonators increasingly reinforce only the fundamental. Listen to Joan

Sutherland or any other coloratura sing variants of the open tube vowel in the Mad Scene from *Lucia di Lammermoor*. It is certainly not simply coincidence that composers set a preponderance of /**a**/ vowels for the coloratura voice.

Marilyn Horne feels that "the highest possible pitch at which a soprano can probably sing decent vowels and words is a G. ... Then you've got to start modifying."[44] Even at G^5 the amount of mouth rounding depends upon the classification and size of the voice, the size of the resonators, the size of the hall, and what kind of music is being sung. For most sopranos, diction is problematical above G^5, and above $B\flat^5$, rounding of the mouth is rarely possible. When singing in the stratosphere, the resonators are small and tightly coupled, the aperture is wide and flat, and projection is possible because of the extremely high tessitura. Johan Sundberg finds that shortening the vocal tract "smoothly and elegantly" is one way of raising the first formant. He goes on to say that the advantage of this method is that f^1 can be raised to higher frequencies than is possible by merely increasing the jaw opening. He does **not** find "that a pitch dependent larynx position is a sign of a poor singing technique ...,"[45] a statement that many methodologies would not condone. Again, form your own opinion by observing great singing on television and by conforming to the acoustical laws concerning cavities.

In the interests of giving aid and reassurance to all harried sopranos, who continually are being castigated for their poor "diction," we offer the following words of comfort. All four authors are eminent and respected members of their professions. The first statement is from a singing teacher, the second is from an acoustician, the third from two researchers in linguistics, and the fourth from a voice scientist.

> The high soprano is the one voice that is justified in choosing the most convenient vowel for her high notes, and using it throughout.[46]

> ... the best sopranos, especially on their higher notes, are prepared to shift formants, deliberately sacrificing vowel accuracy in order to have strong enough low harmonics to make a strong and musical tone.[47]

> For singers who have been discouraged by vain efforts to sing certain vowels at high pitches, it may be a comfort to learn that it is theoretically impossible. This should also be a warning to the music teacher who literally expects "the impossible" from a student![48]

> ... the vowels /a:/, /i:/, and /u:/ were all produced with very similar tongue shapes ... at the fundamental frequency of 960 Hz (pitch B♭^{5}).[49]

Vowel Modification and Intelligibility

Modified vowels are often more intelligible than pure vowels. That statement is difficult for singers to believe. What they "know" cognitively interferes with what they feel, and they logically cannot believe that altered vowels sound anything like the spoken word. Probably the most effective way of allaying their fears is to have them listen to other singers whose voices resemble theirs in size and weight. Those singers who use the ***mezza tinta*** or half-tinted vowel with skill and muscular understanding of how it should feel are surely on the way to vocal longevity. They obtain greater results for less effort. Again we quote Johan Sundberg:

> Since formant frequencies determine vowel quality, shifting the first formant frequency arbitrarily according to pitch might be expected to produce a distorted vowel sound, even an unintelligible one. It does not have this effect. ... If a singer raises her first formant frequency with the pitch, some of that rise is actually required just to maintain the identity of the vowel.[50]

The same concept was similarly stated by a respected teacher and singer fifty years earlier:

> The modification of the vowels ... does not injure or make indistinct our pronunciation. ... On the contrary, the obedience to the natural laws of singing, which causes the slight modification, is alone possible if we accept this doctrine, and the result will be far more natural and spontaneous and true to laws of pronunciation.[51]

Slight shifts in first formant frequencies in particular seem to have a strong effect upon the degree of intelligibility. An example of this kind of vowel shading is shown in Figure 45.

We already have explored the intelligibility versus quality dilemma of the high female voice in some detail. Nelson and Tiffany reported in a 1968 issue of the *NATS Bulletin* that intelligibility declined from 75% to 25% between C^5 and G^5.[52] In 1980 Smith and Scott found substantially the same results, but when transitional cues (consonants) were added to vowels, intelligibility at F^5 was very close to that at C^5.[53] The appropriate use of consonants greatly increases intelligibility. It is hoped that further study of vowel-consonant interaction at specific pitches and dynamic levels is being done. Certainly we all are aware that some singers are much more "understandable" than others, and generally not because they move their mouths more. Articulation of consonants is a subject that deserves infinitely more attention than it has received to date. For a detailed exploration of consonant articulation, Berton Coffin's "Articulation for Opera, Oratorio, and Recital" is highly recommended.[54]

There obviously are important and complex muscular responses required for effective diction in singing. Yet many of the research studies use only one to four subjects or else a group of subjects from a single voice studio. Regardless of how rigorous the procedural controls are, the validity of conclusions from such studies must be open to question.

Although it may be difficult to gather enough trained singers with different methods of voice production at the same time and in the same place, scientific validity surely would be better served by using more than a half-dozen subjects.

The cause of intelligibility, to say nothing of vocal health, has not been well served by the overwhelming majority of post-1950 compositions. In 1890, Morell MacKenzie said:

> Defects in pronunciation ... are very often more justly chargeable to the composer than to the singer, as, from ignorance of the laws as to the pitch of vowels, syllables are associated with notes on which they cannot be properly sounded.[55]

Few composers seem to have read, either then or now, professional and scientific books and journals with precise and detailed information about the fixed formant law and its effect upon intelligibility. Female singers are most at risk, of course, if they are asked to sing /**i**/ and /**e**/ vowels on very high pitches. Much too often syllabic rather than melismatic passages are found at high tessituras. At least on a melisma there is some chance of altering the vowel enough to keep from choking. When Franz Schubert set male texts, he used appropriate vowels on high pitches, e.g., in *Auf dem Strom.* Mozart and Handel were masters at writing for specific voice classifications. They learned by listening. Sopranos should not try to sing Benjamin Britten's *Winter Words.* It was written for Peter Pears, a tenor. These comments are not meant to denigrate in any way contemporary compositional techniques. That is not the point. The point is that the singing voice is not tuned the same as a clarinet or a piano. A composer who wants to write for the voice should first learn how it works.

Vowel Modification and Dynamic Level

Judging from empirical observation, the louder the tone, the more vowel modification is needed. Much of the intensity of a sound is determined by the degree of vocal fold resistance to the air stream, which results in a certain amplitude of movement. The greater the amplitude, the richer the sound spectrum in overtones. A correspondingly larger resonator is needed to accommodate such a sound wave without the tone becoming harsh. Do your own observing the next time an opera is telecast. Note the difference in the mouth opening and vowel coloring for fortissimo and piano singing.

It should be noted that vowel modifications differ with the kind of resonance and phonatory mix employed. For instance, a fully hooked-up voice uses more vocalis activity even at higher frequencies than does a more mixed voice, i.e., one with more "loft" or high mechanism in it. The latter production also requires less vowel modification than the fuller or bigger voice. Berton Coffin remarks that "a voice feels heavy when there is too much low in the voice and feels free when the lower resonance is just right to allow a great deal of the high frequencies 'to pass'."[56] It seems probable that the best resonance possible (superposition) encourages flow phonation and less breath pressure, promotes an easier vocal fold function, and requires a lesser degree of modification. A discussion of the *voix mixte*, a particular kind of register management, is included in Chapter 8.

The Mirror Image

If vowel modification for male and female voices is not alike, and we have presented acoustical reasons to support this statement, what is the principal difference between male and female modifications? Male voices close as they ascend and female voices open. The statement may be oversimplified, but as a basic guide it is valid. As the male voice approaches the passaggio area between E^4 and G^4, the closed vowels /**i**/, /**y**/ and /**u**/ are optimal, depending, of course, on individual differences of voice size and dynamic level. In the highest area of the tenor and baritone voices, a more open embouchure is needed. In master classes recorded in Italy, Luciano Pavarotti assessed the matter in an empirical, rather than scientific, way:

> A tenor normally starts to cover his notes or better to "focus" on F, F♯, and G, and it is usually a forced and unnatural sound which a young man finds hard to believe in, but it is a sound which technically and anatomically speaking produces in the voice a rest for the vocal cords, which will then be ready when the voice goes higher, to vibrate with greater elasticity and therefore enables the notes to be taken which are B♭, B and C, the most difficult notes for a tenor.[57]

This statement is another confirmation of Vennard's belief that by learning the shaping of the resonators, we are unconsciously training the vocal cords. Pavarotti, like all tenors, finds it almost impossible to hear his sound at this tessitura because of increased pharyngeal vibration and high air pressure. Yet he recognizes the feeling of an optimal resonance bore and its influence on top voice singing. Acoustical distuning in this very important bridge area often is the reason why the top notes are only shouts or barks, if they are there at all.

The female singer, on the other hand, closes as the voice descends to conform to the lowering f^1 vowel formants. We have discussed at some length the necessity to open the resonance tract as the female voice goes higher. The f^1 vowel formants move from closed to open as they ascend until only variants of /**a**/ are possible.

As the male voice descends, it uses more open vowels until at the bottom of the range, all vowels become open tube ones. This phenomenon is not scientifically explainable, but is verified by the evidence of tonal spectra taken at that tessitura. It is verifiable empirically, of course, by aural and visual observation. In the middle male range of C^3 to C^4, individual anatomical differences in the resonance tract, in voice classification, and in voice size seem to have a bearing on the degree of opening, but in general the use of half-tinted vowels results in a clearer quality.

In the matter of vowel coloring, the voice is a mirror image, moving from the most closed vowels at approximately F^4 to increasingly open vowels as the sung tone moves away from that central point in either direction.

Speaking and Singing

"Singing is no different than speaking."

How often have you heard that statement? It is difficult to refute a concept which sounds so logical, particularly if it is delivered authoritatively. The reasons for making such a statement are understandable. A singer or a group of singers may be indulging in lazy diction habits. Or the listener may feel that if only the vowels and consonants were articulated more precisely, the text would be more intelligible.

The fact is that good diction is possible, at least in "classical" singing, only after a certain degree of technical proficiency is attained. Vowels make up 99% of the singing sound and must be properly tuned to produce an even, fluid sound. The functional unity of proper breathing, an efficiently operating vibrator (vocal folds), and a well-tuned resonating tract are the prerequisites for the fine art of intelligible diction.

As for singing being no different from speaking, there are certain ways in which it differs greatly.

(1) **Speech is not tied to specific tonal intervals.** In speech there is widespread use of gliding pitch modulations. In singing, though, at least in classical singing, specific tonal steps are indicated, and even slight irregularities of intonation are aesthetically displeasing.

(2) **Speech is not sustained.** Because speech sounds generally are not sustained, the resonators can be quickly adjusted for projection of specific vowels and consonants.

(3) **Formants and the speaking voice.** The ranges of almost all normal adult speaking voices are much lower than those of singing voices. There are no "high C" speakers. The median speaking frequency for males is approximately 145 cps (D^3) and for females approximately 230 cps ($B\flat^3$),[58] both well below the lowest first formant, even allowing for variations in inflection.

(4) **The speaking range is much shorter.** The speaking range seldom encompasses more than a fifth, whereas the singing range is at least two octaves. As a result, in speech there is ample choice of partials for vowel differentiation. This choice, together with swift movement of the articulators to properly alter the resonators (#2 above), gives speech its intelligibility and precision, while the high frequencies common in singing require modifications of the vowels used and changes in normal articulatory speech habits.

(5) **Subglottic pressure and laryngeal positioning.** In speaking, subglottic pressure is used mainly for loudness control; a rise in loudness means a rise in fundamental frequency. In singing, however, "each note requires its own pressure" for the intended loudness **and** pitch.[59] In other words, an increase in loudness does not

> necessarily mean a rise in fundamental frequency. Of equal importance is the fact that the singing formant is seldom present in a speaking voice and consequently the position of the larynx is not significant.

Few speakers, however, can emotionally stir the listener with sheer sound. There are not many like Richard Burton who had the range, the projection, and the palette of colors that our great singers have. Most speech does not need such projection, and indeed, as mentioned above, few speaking voices use the singing formant which provides so much ring to the sound. If the trained singer uses efficient phonation, i.e., the lowest possible amount of heat and friction in the laryngeal area, optimum conversion of breath energy into acoustic power will take place. The conversion rate ranges from 1% to 10% of the energy provided.[60] In contrast, typical conversational speech converts only 0.1%.

Good diction is a laudable and necessary goal for the singer, but is not attained simply by imitating the speaking voice.

The Pure Vowel

> The pure singing or tone vowel is not at all pure in the ordinary sense of the word. ... It is possible to sing twenty different e, i, ah, o, oo's which in their own nature, already mixed, sound pure and intelligible in the word.[61]

It is hoped that Lilli Lehmann's view of pure vowels, written in 1902, is now more understandable than it would have been before reading this chapter. The subject of fixed vowel formants is not easy to understand, but it is crucial to a complete understanding of the singing instrument.

Vowel modification is the practical application of an acoustical law. The implications of that law for the teaching of singing have appeared in the writings of respected pedagogs and scientists from Helmholtz to the present. Implicit in all their investigations is the belief that the singing voice must be "tuned" properly or its functional unity will be seriously impaired.

It seems clear that good breath support, although an essential ingredient of beautiful singing, cannot solve all vocal problems. Force is not a viable substitute for optimum sympathetic resonance. As one young singer declared triumphantly: "Loud is not loudness; loud is projection."

NOTES

1. Johan Sundberg, "The Voice as a Sound Generator," *Research Aspects on Singing* (Stockholm: Royal Swedish Academy of Music, 1981), 7.

2. Appelman, op. cit., 126.

3. Gunilla Carlsson and Johan Sundberg, "Formant Frequency Tuning in Singing," *Journal of Voice*, 6:3 (1992), 256.

4. Sundberg, "Acoustics of the Singing Voice," op. cit., 82.

5. Ibid., 82-83 and 86. See also Peter B. Denes and Elliot N. Pinson, *The Speech Chain* (Garden City, NY: Anchor Press, 1973), 83.

6. Johan Sundberg, "Vocal Tract Resonance in Singing," *NATS Journal*, 44:4 (1988), 12.

7. Ibid.

8. Berton Coffin, "The Singer's Diction," *NATS Bulletin*, 20:3 (1964), 10.

9. Benade, op. cit., 374.

10. Paget, op. cit., 214.

11. C. J. Darwin and R. B. Garner, "Mistuning a Harmonic of a Vowel: Grouping and Phase Effects of Vowel Quality," *Journal of Acoustical Society of America*, 79:3 (1986), 838-845.

12. Sundberg, "The Voice as a Sound Generator," op. cit., 13.

13. Eiji Yanagisawa, Jo Estill, Steven T. Kmucha, and Steven B. Leder, "The Contribution of Aryepiglottic Constriction to 'Ringing' Voice Quality--a Videolaryngoscopic Study with Acoustic Analysis," *Journal of Voice*, 3:4 (1989), 348.

14. Ibid., 350.

15. Sundberg, *Science of Singing Voice*, op. cit., 118-119.

16. Johan Sundberg, "Articulatory Interpretation of the Singing Formant," *Journal of Acoustical Society of America*, 55:4 (1974), 843.

17. Gerrit Bloothooft and Reiner Plomp, "The Sound Level of the Singer's Formant in Professional Singing," *Journal of the Acoustical Society of America*, 79:6 (1986), 2028-2033.

18. Sundberg, "Vocal Tract Resonance," op. cit., 14.

19. Ibid., 15.

20. Martin Rothenberg, "The Voice Source in Singing," *Research Aspects on Singing* (Stockholm: Royal Swedish Academy of Music, 1981), 19.

21. Sundberg, "Acoustics of the Singing Voice," op. cit., 89.

22. Pierre Delattre, "Vowel Color and Voice Quality." *NATS Journal*, 15:1 (1958), 5.

23. Ingo Titze, "Messa di voce," *NATS Journal*, 48:3 (1992), 24.

24. Maureen Stone, Kathleen A. Morrish, Barbara C. Sonies, and Thomas H. Shawker, "Tongue Curvature: A Model of Shape during Vowel Production," *Folia Phoniatrica*, 39 (1987), 308 and 314.

25. Ingo Titze, "Rules for Modifyinging Vowels," *NATS Bulletin*, 40:3 (1984), 30.

26. Fant, op. cit., 64.

27. T. Chiba and M. Kajiyama, *The Vowel* (Tokyo: Phonetic Society of Japan, 1958), 154.

28. Titze, "Rules," op. cit., 30.

29. Sundberg, "Vocal Tract Resonance," op. cit., 12-13.

30. Fant, op. cit., 219.

31. Ibid., 160.

32. Sundberg, "Vocal Tract Resonance," op. cit., 18.

33. Berton Coffin, *Sounds of Singing* (Metuchen, NJ: Scarecrow Press, 1987), 57.

34. Sundberg, "Acoustics of the Singing Voice," op. cit., 84.

35. Vennard, *Singing*, op. cit., p. 80.

36. Martin Rothenberg, "Acoustic Reinforcement of Vocal Fold Vibratory Behavior in Singing," Chapter 34, *Vocal Physiology*, Osamu Fujimura, ed., op. cit., 386.

37. Coffin, *Overtones*, op. cit., 171.

38. Ingo Titze, "Some Thoughts on Source-System Interdependence," *NATS Journal*, 38:5 (1982), 28.

39. Titze and Sundberg, "Vocal Intensity," op. cit., 2946.

40. Gunnar Fant, "Glottal Flow: Models & Interaction," *Journal of Phonetics*, 14:3/4 (1986), 393-399.

41. Benade, op. cit., 80.

42. Sundberg, "Acoustics of the Singing Voice," op. cit., 89.

43. Johan Sundberg, "Studies of the Soprano Voice," *Journal of Research in Singing*, 1:1 (1977), 25-35.

44. Quoted in Jerome Hines, *Great Singers on Great Singing*, (Garden City, NY: Doubleday, 1982), 142.

45. Johan Sundberg, "Supralaryngeal Contributions to Vocal Loudness and Projection," *Care of the Professional Voice*, 13th Symposium, Part 1, Van Lawrence, ed. (NY: The Voice Foundation, 1984), 204-205.

46. Vennard, *Singing*, op. cit., 159.

47. Hall, op. cit., 332-333.

48. Howie and Delattre, op. cit., 8.

49. Sundberg, "Vocal Tract Resonance," op. cit., 17-18.

50. Sundberg, "Acoustics of the Singing Voice," op. cit., 90.

51. Herbert Witherspoon, *Singing* (New York: G. Schirmer, 1925; reprint by DaCapo, 1980), 30.

52. Howard D. Nelson and William R. Tiffany, "The Intelligibility of Song," *NATS Bulletin*, 25:2 (1968), 28.

53. Lloyd A. Smith and Brian L. Scott, "Increasing the Intelligibility of Sung Vowels," *Journal of the Acoustical Society of America*, 67:5 (1980), 1797.

54. Berton Coffin, *Historical Vocal Pedagogy Classics*, (Metuchen, NJ: Scarecrow Press, 1989), Appendix F.

55. MacKenzie, op. cit., 105.

56. Coffin, *Overtones*, op. cit., 200.

57. Pavarotti, op. cit., Mizar record.

58. Figures from John Askill, *Physics of Musical Sounds* (New York: D. Van Nostrand, 1979), 148.

59. Johan Sundberg, "What's So Special about Singers?" *Journal of Voice*, 4:2 (1990), 108.

60. Ingo Titze, "Is There a Scientific Explanation for Tone Focus and Voice Placement?" *NATS Bulletin*, 37:5 (1981), 27.

61. Lehmann, op. cit., 60.

Chapter 8

VOCAL REGISTERS

The subject of vocal registers continues to be controversial. Are there registers at all? If so, how many? Where do they occur? What causes registers and how can they be blended? The singer can feel and hear certain changes in his/her vocal production, but each teacher seems to have a different explanation for what is happening and how to deal with it. "No other area of vocal instruction is as shrouded with mystery, semantic confusion, and controversy as the subject of registers and registration."[1]

To answer the first question, yes, registers do exist. There is unanimity in the scientific community and a strong majority opinion among singing teachers. Generally those pedagogs who disagree believe that an uneven scale is only the result of "poor technique," not of physiological factors. Yet what is poor technique if not physiological dysfunction? Vocal registers probably are not "removed" in the literal sense of that word, but their effects are blended or equalized until they are no longer apparent to the discriminating ear (and the singer's throat).

What is a vocal register? Garcia (1894)[2] and Colton (1988)[3] have similar short definitions.

> A register is a series of consecutive homogeneous sounds produced by one mechanism, differing essentially from another series of sounds equally homogeneous produced by another mechanism ...
>
> A register is a series of consecutive fundamental frequencies of approximately equal quality.

The inclusive nature of the first definition suited what was proven knowledge about registers then, and it apparently suits that knowledge today.

It seems very probable, considering scientific evidence **AND** empirical observation, that the two key factors concerning registers are (1) the use of air, particularly subglottic air pressure changes, and (2) resonance coupling and its effect on the sound wave. These factors easily encompass multiple views about the nature of vocal registers.

Vennard believed that the matter of registers is primarily myoelastic,[4] i.e., is muscular and is the result of vibratory patterns of the intrinsic muscles of the larynx coordinated with subglottic pressure. Hollien (1982) felt that "a voice register is a totally laryngeal event. ..."[5], an idea which he tried to support with perceptual, acoustical, physiological, and aerodynamic data. He also was pursuing studies of resonance-based quality changes and hoped to overlay the results on his laryngeal model. Lehmann maintained that poor vowels (resonance) cause registers,[6] as did MacKenzie, who felt that "the difference between artistic and inartistic production of the voice depends far more on the management of the resonators than on the adjustment of the vocal cords."[7] Shakespeare, on the other hand, emphasized the importance of the suspensory network of extrinsic muscles when he said that "registers seem to be influenced by different sets of placing muscles which balance the larynx in the exact position necessary to any note."[8]

Apparently blending the registers is not possible merely through attention to limited and specific areas of the vocal mechanism. A gestalt or total functional unit composed of respiration, phonation, and resonation is needed.

How many Registers?

Vocal registers are a physiological fact. Questions still persist, though, about the number of registers, their nature, and their training.

Traditional names for registers are still used in the voice studio with such terms as "head," "chest," and "middle."

They are based on singers' sensations. Although inference, imagery, and sensation are used successfully in many voice studios, their use seems to be more effective if the teacher understands the physiological meaning of these traditional terms. For example, the quality of the lower register does ***not*** emanate from the chest, as was pointed out in the section on possible auxiliary resonators in Chapter 6. Nor does the mechanism of the upper register depend solely upon resonation in the sinuses, head or "mask." It seems unlikely that new generic terms will replace the traditional ones, however. It is extremely difficult to banish traditions.

A committee of eminent physicians and scientists found the traditional terms extremely subjective and "illogical if not absurd,"[9] and identified the following registers.

(1) The very lowest register (traditional terms: pulse, growl)
(2) The register where most speaking and singing occur (traditional terms: modal, heavy)
(3) A high register used primarily for singing and rarely for speaking (traditional terms: falsetto, light)
(4) A very high register found only in women and children (traditional terms: whistle, flute)

An additional register in the middle of the frequency range the committee found difficult to define scientifically, but concluded that "it receives so much (subjective) support, it cannot be ignored."[10] This register is an important problem area in the training of female singers and is traditionally called middle.

If one disregards the growl and the flute mechanisms, two primary registers remain of those listed by the committee of scientists. Both of these registers are determined primarily by laryngeal function. Thus this view of vocal registers reaffirms what has been the prevailing opinion for the past twenty-five years: the primary influence on registers is laryngeal.

This concept implies a complex synergy of vocal fold function and subglottic pressure. The two registers are variously termed light-heavy or upper-lower. Vennard proposes a hypothesis of two registers which he calls "light mechanism" and "heavy mechanism."[11] His terminology is based upon laryngeal function, but he also maintains that these two registers can overlap by an octave, which can be sung in either laryngeal adjustment. Thus he accounts for that difficult "middle" area mentioned earlier.

Heavy and light laryngeal behavior is contrasted below.

Heavy	*Light*
thick cords	thin cords
wide amplitude	narrower amplitude
firm glottal closure	brief and/or incomplete glottal closure
rich in partials	fewer partials
vocalis active	crico-thyroid active

Most of these elements have been discussed in earlier chapters. The coordination of intrinsic laryngeal muscles is particularly important for a smooth transition over the laryngeal bridge area (approximately E^4 or F^4). In heavy mechanism the isometric contraction of the vocalis is strong. As the action of the crico-thyroid increases and vocalis decreases, the vocal folds become longer and thinner. They tend to gap in the middle (medial) area so the lateral crico-arytenoid adductors must pull more strongly. All of this joint action is only possible if the larynx itself is stabilized in a comfortably low position by the extrinsic suspensory muscles. In addition to all that, the assistance of appropriate breath management adds the proper air flow-subglottic pressure ratio.

The importance of air flow-pressure ratios was discussed at some length under **Matching Formants and the Harmonic Series** in Chapter 7. Hill believes that "the increase of air flow over the passaggio will facilitate the coordination of the two registers."[12] He is probably referring here to the laryngeal bridge, but the same coordination is required on all major register bridges, be they physiological or acoustical in nature. Almost all singers have experienced an increase in pressure and air flow as pitch rises until the highest frequency of a given register is reached. At this point, especially in the early stages of training, the mechanism shifts to a lower pressure-flow ratio. Many choral musicians call this phenomenon the "lift of the breath," which is certainly descriptive of what is probably a decrease in acoustical loading on the vocal folds.

If the vocalis adjusts to the increasing action of the crico-thyroid as the voice ascends, the register transition takes place smoothly. If not, the transition is sudden, jerky, and completely different in quality. For males, the shift at this bridge is from chest to falsetto, two very different qualities unless adjustment has been made for the male *voix mixte.* This subject will be discussed further in the section on male registers. For females, the shift is from chest to middle voice, but if the vocalis has not permitted increased crico-thyroid action, there is a "break" into the pure head voice instead of a smooth transition into the female *voix mixte.* This jerky transition often is heard when female singers belt too high. More about this transition is found in the secton on female registers. For both males and females, singing with too much heavy mechanism in too high a range can cause vocal fatigue and measurably shorten the life of a voice.

In his excellent summary of register terminology, Timberlake (1990)[13] cites the Vennard register model described above as well as the names used by the Lampertis, two of the foremost singing teachers of the 19th and early 20th centuries, and those used by Johan Sundberg, today's leading acoustician of the singing voice. Both Lampertis used the three-register model of chest, medium or mixed, and head for both sexes. In contrast, Sundberg prefers modal and falsetto for males and chest, medium and head for females. How curious that he uses scientific terms for male singers and empirical or experience-based ones for female singers.

Although the bulk of scientific literature on registers emphasizes the laryngeal adjustment, there recently has been more interest in the effects of shifts in partials and formant enhancement. Semantically, some scientists prefer to call these resonance adjustments acoustic/timbre events rather than registers. The fact is that most singers "feel" only one register bridge in the larynx, the one at about 300 cps. They talk about "that funny clicking feeling down here" (pointing to the larynx). Otherwise, the more muscularly sophisticated singers use a variety of kinesthetic comments to describe articulatory problems in the vocal tube, which to them is like a sound speaker whose baffles are out of line.

During the panel discussion at the 1980 Care of the Professional Voice Symposium, Large suggested that although some registers are laryngeally determined, the bridge between female middle and head registers is acoustically determined, as is the one between the male chest and head registers.[14] He went on to say that the latter transition appears to be accomplished by reinforcing the fundamental frequency with the first formant. Titze objected to this inclusion of acoustic determinants in register definition because he felt it then would be impossible to establish relations in the "chain among physiological bases, acoustical bases and perceptual bases."[15] Yet the voice is not solely a physiological mechanism, but also an acoustical one. Perhaps for the scientist these events can be considered separately. For the singer and the singing teacher, they cannot. If this difference of opinion is merely a semantic one, that is understandable. If it is a functional one, its rationale is in error. The physiological function of the vocal folds and the acoustic properties of the resonance tract are inter-dependent, as Titze himself points out so clearly in the following statement. "The vocal tract acts as an acoustic load on the vocal folds, thereby dictating in varying degrees what the vocal folds can or cannot do."[16] Oncley suggests the use of "mechanism change" to describe laryngeal adjustments and "shifts in formant position" to describe acoustic adjustments.[17] Whatever the terminology, many singing teachers subscribe to the realistic pedagogical approach of three registers. So did Manuel Garcia, a great teacher, and Enrico Caruso, a great singer. Although a relatively new concept to voice scientists, vocal-tract-related registers have received increasing attention in the past ten years.

Where do registers occur? It is often easiest to identify them by means of the transition or "lift" areas mentioned earlier when an increase in light mechanism seems to occur. Arnold makes a fascinating analogy between these shifts in the singing voice and an automobile gear ratio.

> The natural transition between two adjacent registers may be compared to the gearshift of a car. ... The same absolute vehicle speed can be maintained by driving either with high rpm in low gear or by fewer engine revolutions in the next higher gear. Driving with the minimal amount of gas flow at a given speed is the most economical manner with regard to gas consumption and engine conservation.[18]

If the interplay of forces in the singing voice is used judiciously, maximum smoothness and blend of registers will produce optimum breath flow, optimum resonation and optimum vocal health. The belter who pushes his/her sound with high revolutions per minute in low gear is risking permanent damage to the vocal engine.

The location of register bridges or passaggi is still a subject of scientific and pedagogical controversy. It is instructive to note, though, that as a voice grows in size and in focus, intonation problems generally occur first at these bridges.

The Female Registers

The three main female registers are chest, middle, and head. The whistle or flute is considered an auxiliary register. Some authorities feel that the middle register is not a separate register, but an overlapping of the chest (heavy) and head (light). Subjective as it may be, however, actual vocal experience reveals three registers, each of which exhibits distinct differences in tone quality.

Mathilde Marchesi (1821-1913) studied four years with Manuel Garcia and subsequently became the most successful teacher of female singers in the history of vocal pedagogy. Among her students were Nellie Melba (Australian), Emma Calve (French), Emma Eames (American), Ilma di Murska (Croatian), and Etelka Gerster (Hungarian). She herself was German, but her teaching embodied the traditions of Italian eighteenth-century *bel canto* singing. No wonder then that pedagogs and researchers alike have studied Marchesi's ideas about female registration. Although she attributed the phenomenon of registers to the resonators and did not recognize changing vibrational modes of the vocal folds as a factor, her teaching record is evidence of the validity of her aural perceptions. Among contemporary singers, Marilyn Horne, Joan Sutherland, and Monserrat Caballé all agree with her model of the female registers.[19]

For the chest register the vocal folds are full and broad. They vibrate over their entire breadth and billow from side to side in a waving motion. Marchesi says the highest note that should be sung in chest voice varies between E^4 and $F\sharp^4$.[20] Vennard says the chest voice should be taken no higher than F^4, with D^4 preferable. He goes on to say that although it does no harm for a man to develop his falsetto downward, "forcing the female chest voice upwards is dangerous if not actually malpractice."[21] Strong words, but justified because such a practice can be as harmful as the heavy glottal attack.

As the pitch rises, the opposition of the crico-thyroid to the vocalis increases, the cords begin to elongate and tense, and only the edges of the folds vibrate on an almost parallel course. In blending chest and middle registers, breath pressure must be slightly decreased to go over the bridge or else a strong vocal contraction will bring back the heavy chest resonance. At the same time, in order to prevent a sudden decrease in dynamic level on the first notes of the middle register, an extra surge of breath is helpful. This kind of breath management is noticeable in the training of young voices, and a rather breathy sound is common at first. Marchesi has words of advice about handling resonance factors when moving between these two registers. To equalize the scale, slightly close the last two chest notes when ascending.[22] As the ability to balance resonance and breathing factors improves, the tone will become clear and focused. Undue weight and/or volume is not helpful and will only produce a more noticeable transition. Perceptual research studies of the female middle register show that it is not as easily identified as chest/modal or head/falsetto in function, yet the results are statistically greater than chance so its existence cannot be dismissed out of hand. Many singing teachers find irrefutable empirical evidence of its existence. Garcia believes it extends from C^4 to C^5, and only the lowest third can be sung in either chest or middle register.[23] It often has a somewhat veiled or breathy quality and if the back vowels are dull, they can be alternated with ringing front vowels to increase their brilliance. Garcia also thinks that weakness in the middle register can be attributed to abuse of the chest register.[24] He certainly would applaud the advice of Dr. Brodnitz.[25]

> Ideal singing is done in a mixture of register characteristics--a voix mixte. Each tone of the compass receives a little of the color of the opposing registers. ... The only case where a pure register is used in perfect singing is the coloratura, who sings in a clear head register.

No singing teacher or voice scientist has found as clear a definition of *voix mixte* as the one above.

In a direct quote attributed to his famous voice teacher, Giovanni Battista Lamperti, William Earl Brown uses this apt analogy.

> You do not water a tree at the top but at the roots--and the tree spreads and blooms as a natural consequence. It is the proper training of the middle voice that brings the beautiful head voice.[26]

The middle voice is an area of prime importance for the female singer, and it is only after she learns how to manage this part of her range that real vocal development begins.

For the pure head voice, the action of the crico-thyroid stretchers is reinforced by additional palatal lift. The chink of the glottis is open slightly and the epiglottis is fully raised. Air flow increases. The result is a light, soaring sound with minimal overtones. When the antagonistic actions of the extrinsic stylo-pharyngeal system against the major depressors and the vocalis against the crico-thyroid are increased, the vocal folds adduct more firmly, their amplitude increases, and breath energy must be deepened. The louder the tone, the more the vocalis works and the greater the breath energy needed. The larynx stays comfortably low and the ventricular cavities (located just above the "true" vocal folds) widen. The result is the full, "hooked-up" head voice and a sound wave rich in upper partials. Again Manuel Garcia anticipated the results of 20th century acoustical research when he said that "the volume of sound depends on the expansion of the pharynx and of the vestibule of the larynx."[27] Arnold Rose adds that by using head voice it is possible to sing for a longer time without tiring, and to use higher intensities without damaging the cords.[28]

The highest note in the middle register is F^5, although Garcia indicates that the interval between $C\#^5$ and E^5 includes the "blending notes" which form the bridge between the middle and head registers.[29] These latter notes are difficult to tune and frequently are a sign of changes in tessitura and/or voice size when intonation problems appear in a previously well-tuned voice. The larger the voice the greater is the need for proper vowel modification in this bridge area. In other words, first formants **must** reinforce the fundamental frequency.

For example, the /**e**/ vowel is shaded toward /ε/, the /**i**/ migrates toward /**e**/ or even /ε/ in bigger voices, the /**o**/ absorbs some of the /ɔ/ vowel, and the /**u**/ modifies to /ʊ/, /**o**/, or /ɔ/, depending upon voice size, classification, style, ascending or descending line, and other pertinent factors. As the frequency rises from F^4 to these bridge notes between the middle and head registers, the vowels must open to match the fundamental. Refer to the charts of first formant frequencies on pages 150 and 152. Both female and male voices are narrow at F^4.

> I think the voice has a shape wider at the top and bottom and narrower in the middle. The middle is where the danger area is, around E flat, E, and F. I almost never carry the chest sound above F and because of this I can get from one register to another without difficulty.[30]

Flawless intonation probably is easier to achieve for the smaller voices than for the big dramatic ones. Pleasants says that all of Marchesi's students had "an absolutely even scale, a lightness and precision of attack, an absence of any kind of forcing, an immaculate intonation, even in the most rapid passages, and a marvelous ease at the upper extreme of the vocal compass."[31] These voices were ideal for the light, florid music of Rossini, Donizetti, or even Massenet. Their singing lives undoubtedly were longer than those of their contemporaries, but they did not sing Verdi or Wagner. Melba even refused to learn *Madama Butterfly*.

Among today's young female singers, the head register often is underused and sometimes rejected entirely. Much of the popular music is written in low keys, and chest register is carried up well beyond F^4. It is a classic example of too much effort being expended on the upper notes of a given register, making it impossible to develop any power on the low notes of the next register. Remedial work is tediously slow, and there is a long period when the sound is fuzzy in both registers. The full compass of the voice and the colors required for varying emotions are not attainable when the singer commands only one register and one quality.

The light head voice mix requires less vowel modification than the full head voice, although even this relatively "pure" sound cannot tolerate the closed front vowels on F^5, $F\sharp^5$, and G^5 without certain alterations. Much depends upon individual differences in vocal size and weight. For the full head voice, slight rounding at the passaggio plus the addition of /ʌ/ or /œ/ often succeeds best. Above G^5, variations of /**a**/ must be used, again depending upon personal vocal characteristics. Rounding above $B\flat^5$ is not advised except in rare cases, generally by the highest coloraturas.

The whistle or flute register, which usually begins about C^6, was first recognized by Leopold Mozart. The sound is similar to that of a recorder or piccolo, appears to be almost entirely sinusoidal, and under analysis has very few upper partials. Zemlin (1988) describes this register as:[32]

> ... a laryngeal whistle which does not seem to be produced by the vibration of the vocal folds but by the whistling escape of air between them.

The cords are completely damped except for the flow of air through the small oval opening. Subglottic pressure is very high, about 30 cm H_2O.[33] A fairly high air flow may be needed initially for the singer to find her flute register; adjustments in air flow can be made when she becomes more accustomed to the effortlessness of that kind of production. Once a singer experiences this register, she is amazed at how easy the production is. Air flow also decreases measurably as the head and whistle registers become more blended.

Although the dynamic level of the sound is low, the projection is excellent because of the very high frequencies.

The report of the Committee on Vocal Registers at the 12th Symposium on Care of the Professional Voice (1983) concluded that the whistle register is not particularly relevant to singing.[34] Perhaps that perception comes from their observation of female singers who have successfully achieved a mix of head and whistle resonance. Based on first hand observation of concert and opera performances and upon practical experience in the studio, we cannot agree. Many singers, both sopranos and mezzo-sopranos, do not handle the upper range with ease and agility, regardless of what that range is. The tone sounds stiff and the vibrato is uneven. A legato is impossible. If the whistle register is used in vocalizing, however, there often is a marked improvement. Coffin feels that this register is helpful in extending the upper range. Furthermore, he contends that it blends into the head voice to produce the true dramatic coloratura. Without it, only the light coloratura is possible.[35]

The Male Registers

The three primary male registers are chest, head, and falsetto. In such male voices as the low bass, the total range is sung in chest register, and in all male voices a larger portion of the range consists of chest register than in any of the female voice types.

Garcia maintains that the chest timbre extends to D^4 for basses, $E\flat^4$ for baritones, and F^4 or $F\sharp^4$ for tenors, and his estimates are still valid more than a century later.[36] As in the female chest voice, the glottis remains closed for at least 40% of the vibratory cycle, resulting in a rich spectrum of upper overtones.

The male head voice is a blending of heavy and light mechanisms to attain a *voix mixte*, but it has a very different color and projection from that of the female middle voice.

Observable signs of register blending in the bridge or passaggio area are a comfortable low laryngeal position (use of the extrinsic strap muscles), elevation of the soft palate, generally a more closed and rounded mouth position, somewhat darker vowels, and increased air flow. All these signs indicate that so-called "covered" singing is based on increased resonance within the widened resonance tract. If this kind of cavity coupling and vertical laryngeal positioning are not present, however, the "open" tone that results overloads the vocalis, and the sound either becomes a shout or "breaks." Covered singing, on the other hand, makes full use of the vocalis without causing overcontraction. Early electromyographic (needle electrode) studies by Vennard and Hirano showed that in open singing, vocalis and sterno-hyoid activity decreased rapidly and suddenly with a rise in frequency. In covered singing, however, activity of the crico-thyroid, the vocalis, the lateral crico-arytenoid adductor, and the sterno-hyoid depressor *gradually* increased with a rise in frequency.[37] Almost twenty years later, the traditional signs of covered singing to blend male registers in the passaggio were confirmed, i.e., the widened laryngo-pharynx, the comfortably low larynx, the raised soft palate, the lowering of f^1 via rounded and closed vowels, and increased and constant transglottal air flow.[38] Certainly the recognition of differing transition points for various vowels permits a more gradual adjustment between chest and head voice and the eventual mastery of an even scale.

It is interesting to note that at the opposite pole from the open sound of the raised larynx, Vennard and Hirano found that an excessively low larynx produced even higher muscular exertion in the intrinsic muscles.[39] This kind of position is inefficient as well as vocally tiring because the great increase in dynamic level which is expected does not occur.

The intensity or amplitude of vibration and the multitude of overtones in the sound wave are regulated by a firm glottal closure, the longer length of time the glottis is closed, and the high air pressure used. In laryngeal appearance, this blended head voice resembles the chest register more than it does the falsetto.

The full male head voice extends to B♭^{4} and even to C^5 for those lucky tenors who have a full high C "from the chest." From B♭^{3} to E♭^{4} a gentle rounding of the embouchure often prevents the tone from becoming too thin, although the fully covered, closed vowel should not be used yet. From E^4 to G^4 the following vowels, *appropriately shaded*, are helpful for bridging: /**i**/, /**y**/, /**u**/, /**ø**/, /**o**/, and /**e**/. The first three vowels have f^1 frequencies around 350 cps (F^4), and the latter three are somewhat higher. As the pitch rises, /**I**/, /ʊ/, /**ø**/, /œ/, /**e**/, and /ɛ/ come into play, but specific modification depends upon the size of the voice, the classification, the interval being sung, and the desired coloring. The final arbiter is the ear of the teacher, or the sense of "placement" of the experienced singer. Most vowels will appear in mixed form or ***mezza tinta*** (half colored). Above A^4 the resonance coupling must be extremely tight, forming one large resonator. The open tube vowels, particularly /**Λ**/, are mixed with all other vowels. Above B^4, the /**æ**/ is the vowel of choice. Listen to Pavarotti, Kraus, or any of the tenors who have the high C.

According to Hirano, the major breathing and phonatory characteristics of the falsetto are:[40]

(1) relaxed vocalis muscle
(2) stretched crico-thyroids
(3) incomplete closure along the total length of the vocal ligaments
(4) great increase of air flow
(5) great decrease of air pressure

Although falsetto behavior formerly was thought to be solely the result of the damping of the vocal folds (as in a violin string), some authorities now think extreme longitudinal tension of the folds creates the effect of damping.[41] The tension of the folds creates the effect of damping.[41] The vocalis is almost totally relaxed, while the crico-thyroid is stretched to its maximum. The approximation of the front portions of the thyroid and cricoid cartilages often can be seen or felt in contrast to their more separated position in the chest register. In some falsettos, vibration takes place only along a spindle-shaped opening in the front portion of the cords, while other falsettos exhibit a soft, incomplete closure along the total length of the cords. Reasons for this difference in behavior are not known. Most researchers also find that the vocal folds do not close completely at the back, but leave a glottal chink. Because of all these factors, the glottal closure time is short and often incomplete, the amplitude of the folds is narrow, and there are very few upper partials in the sound wave. There is greater breath flow than in either the male chest or full head registers.

Some pedagogs favor the use of falsetto voice to develop the full head voice, contending that such an approach leads to more ring and avoids the danger of an overly dark and weighty sound. They believe that young voices in particular have difficulty vocalizing only in ascending patterns into the passaggio and above, and that falsetto exercises develop strength in the crico-thyroid stretcher and prevent the vocalis muscle from over-working. Other teachers feel equally strongly that the falsetto has no relation to the full head voice and that its use as a training device leads to a thin, overly-bright sound. The decision must be left to individual teachers and their particular aesthetic preferences.

Those pedagogs who do use the falsetto generally favor descending scales or arpeggios. During this major transition from falsetto to full head voice, there is a sudden closure along the entire vocal fold length, an abrupt decrease in air flow and an increase in subglottic pressure, a much longer closed portion of the oscillatory cycle, and greater vocal fold mass. These events happen very quickly in terms of physiological adjustment. It is helpful if the singer consciously increases air flow volume at the bridge (generally about F^4) to alleviate the effects of such an abrupt decrease in air flow. At the same time, it is unlikely that this aerodynamic compensation will be effective unless the vowel is appropriately altered as well.

An auxiliary male register located below the chest register is variously called straw bass, pulse, fry, or growl register. It sounds a bit like the rustling of straw and is often used in Russian church choirs. Although once considered a voice disorder, in the last 50 years it has been classified as a distinct and normal vocal register. It can extend as low as E^1 (44 cps). Examination of vocal fold function shows a firm closure of the edges of the cords, a very long glottal closure time, minimal air flow, and no change in length with a change in fundamental frequency within its own register.[42] Vocalis activity is completely unopposed; the crico-thyroid is totally at rest.[43] And finally, the ventricular spaces just above the vocal folds are greatly diminished, sometimes even eliminated. Since the false folds are passive, non-muscular masses, could this unusual configuration be an extension of vertical phase behavior? Such a puzzling mixture of characteristics is found in none of the other registers. Research continues.

Although not strictly a matter of register per se, this seems a suitable place for a few words about counter-tenors and falsettists. They are not the same. Falsettists are usually baritones or basses (like Alfred Deller) who have chosen to sing almost exclusively with a reinforced falsetto production.[44] These singers are frequently called counter-tenors, which confuses the matter even more. The true counter-tenor is usually higher in tessitura and sounds fuller than the falsettist. Although such a description is perceptual rather than factual, it is all we have at this time. Almost no research has been done on the falsettist or the counter-tenor, and until we have more physiological and acoustical information, we can only rely on aural perception.

Be he counter-tenor or falsettist, however, the very high male voice has become more accepted as a "legitimate" voice type, owing chiefly to the interest in Baroque and pre-Baroque music and the performance practices of those periods.

It is incumbent upon the dedicated singing teacher to learn as much as possible about the function of this kind of male voice.

Belting

Controversy still rages about the physiology and acoustics of the belting mode of singing and about its effect upon the larynx. Unfortunately, a high percentage of classically trained singing teachers know almost nothing about the mechanics of producing this sound and refuse to even consider teaching anyone who wishes to belt. Consequently, many prospective Broadway or music theatre singers substitute style for a solid vocal technique and never learn how to emit a high intensity sound with as much functional freedom as possible. Brodnitz takes a realistic view of the situation.[45]

> Eight out of 10 students that any singing teacher has in the studio will not wind up on the opera stage, or on the concert. In some form, she or he will be in musicals or in one of these bands. The profession of teaching of singing should develop ideas on how one can deal with students like them.

First of all, one must be flexible, but only within the limits of what a given voice can tolerate, be it training for opera, jazz, musical comedy, or gospel. Sataloff has a marvelous athletic analogy.[46]

> They (rock singers) are always afraid that they will come out sounding like opera singers. I tell them simply: "You are an athlete." Steve Carlton wouldn't be pitching at the age of 40 without a pitching coach. Once you learn how to throw a ball, whether you throw a baseball, a softball, or a basketball is up to you. That's a matter of style. But learning how to use your muscles so that you know where it's going to go when you let go of it is a matter of athletic training.

What is belting? Van Lawrence sets forth the following physical parameters.[47]

(1) modal or speaking voice register extended upward
(2) relatively high amplitudes
(3) tongue base elevated
(4) larynx elevated
(5) narrow pharyngeal diameter
(6) closed ventricular spaces
(7) epiglottis tilted over the larynx

Edwin agrees and suggests that belting is "aggressive and extended lower register or chest voice dominant singing."[48] Estill's research presented at the Ninth Symposium on Care of the Professional Voice in 1980 lists additional characteristics.[49]

(1) a very high energy level
(2) a higher level of vocalis activity than for any other singing mode
(3) higher activity in the extrinsic muscles than for any other singing mode
(4) soft dynamic level not possible
(5) no mixing or coloring with other singing modes

Yet is belting a form of chest voice singing carried up the scale? The excessively long closed phase of the vibratory cycle (Estill estimates as much as 70% over a two-octave range[50]), the high laryngeal position, the reduced air flow, and the absence of vibrato all indicate that it is not. In addition, the operatic chest voice is richest in its low range, but the belt voice thins out down there.

Is there "good" belting and "bad" belting? Perhaps. Unfortunately, we do not know why some singers survive eight shows a week for decades, like the legendary Ethel Merman, and others develop laryngeal pathologies in a relatively short time. It has been our personal perceptual observation that those belters who have sung successfully for a long period of time tend to use a high degree of nasal resonance. Estill describes the sound as "loud, brassy, sometimes nasal, always 'twangy' ..."[51] Miles and Hollien feel that belting "... exhibits little-to-no vibrato but a high level of nasality."[52] Their conclusions are based on their own observations and collation of replies to a survey on belting. Sullivan disagrees and says that nasality is a color choice to be used for interpretation only and then only sparingly because it tires the throat.[53] She provides no physiological explanation of why it is tiring.

It is extremely difficult to separate fact from fiction, cultural conditioning from willingness to experiment. Reputable laryngologists continue to warn us about this kind of singing. They see singers with obvious symptoms of hyperfunctional habits, almost all of which are centered in the throat. Redness and swelling on the vocal ligaments, tender neck muscles, loss of control, and vocal fatigue are a few of the more common warning signs. The same conditions are observed in some classical singers immediately after heavy vocal use. A period of vocal rest follows, whereas that luxury is not available to music theater singers. Or is it possible that belters are more at risk because so few of them undertake a systematic technical regimen? "... it appears well established that the singer who belts frequently experiences vocal pathology. Unfortunately, the reason for this relationship is both poorly understood and subject to controversy."[54]

A great deal of research needs to be done. Central to our understanding of belting is the need to confirm or reject the view that this kind of singing can cause severe vocal fold damage.

(1) Is belting harmful in and of itself?
(2) Does damage occur only if the singer does not do it "correctly?"
(3) Are there some singers who by reason of personality or musical preference are not suited for belting?

(4) Are there some singers with "delicate" throats who are not physiologically suited for belting (or opera, for that matter)?

To the teacher who must deal with belters now and cannot wait for future research studies, take comfort from Robert Edwin's advice. He feels strongly that the singer can be separated from a particular style in order to explore technical matters, and these new insights can then be integrated into a given style to the degree that the style permits.[55]

It is not suggested that teachers abdicate their ethical responsibilities to advocate a healthy vocal technique. It **is** suggested that our profession has a responsibility to all singers, not just to those whose aesthetic preference we agree with.

Blending Registers

At the beginning of this chapter we made only passing reference to the question most frequently asked by singers and singing teachers: How are registers blended? Although any answers are of necessity subjective and dependent upon specific teaching methodology, it would be cowardly to beg the question entirely.

There is no doubt that breath management, laryngeal adjustments, and acoustic factors work together in endless combinations to produce changes in tone quality which are called registers. The scientists want to fit concrete data into a specific "model." They can hear different vocal qualities, and they want to know how these differences come about, what specific mechanisms are used. Voice teachers also need to know as much as possible about what actually happens, but the knowledge does not per se tell them how to help a student sing an even scale. The task of voice teachers is not to isolate the registers, but to make them imperceptible. Singers relate to subjective sensations, to what they feel. Since every single note of a vocal scale must be minutely adjusted because no two are produced exactly alike, singers simply do not have time to intellectualize whether this tone is in middle, that is in chest, or that is altered to a lateral /**o**/. If they do, they become well programmed robots instead of singers. Voice teachers so often use imagery in their teaching because they are trying to understand and to work with what each singer feels. The process is, in the final analysis, an empirical one.

Of the three major functional branches of the singing voice, i.e., breathing, phonation, and resonation, the first and the last are the only ones under the direct control of the singer. Not only is it an abusive practice to try to manipulate the intrinsic muscles of the larynx, it is futile as well. Proper function of the vocal folds is a consequence of breathing and resonance interdependence.

One of the major controversies among voice scientists is whether the term "register" should apply only to laryngeal behavior or to acoustic events as well. Those holding the former view maintain that if the terms "register" and "quality" become interchangeable, there will be no clear definition of either. Advocates of the latter opinion say that it is impossible to functionally separate the overall structure and define what actions belong exclusively to the larynx, to the vocal tract, or to the subglottic system. It seems unlikely that the narrow laryngeally oriented definition of the term "register" will be accepted among singers and teachers of singing, any more than new generic names recommended by the voice scientists. Traditions survive almost as long in the performing arts as in the military.

In light of the physiological interdependence of the singing voice, the vocal tract can be altered in the following ways:

(1) laryngeal positioning
(2) shaping of the oral-pharyngeal cavities by:

a) tongue placement
b) jaw opening
c) embouchure alterations
d) relative tension and lift of the soft palate

To the above controllable changes in the resonating tract must be added voluntary techniques of breath control, sometimes referred to as ***appoggio***, to bring about differing kinds of subglottic air pressure. Slow, even breathing, without holding air back or releasing it in jerky spurts, is needed for skilled control of air pressure. It cannot be too strongly stated that excessive breath pressure is an inefficient and dangerous substitute for amplification of sound by means of optimum resonance. Although it is true that increased breath pressure is needed for a crescendo, there definitely is a point of no return when the articulators become rigid and the tone is more like a shout than a singing sound. Excessive air pressure is all too often the culprit.

Thus all three factors, air management, laryngeal positioning, and resonance coupling combine to determine register events and eventual register blending.

Many authors agree that loud phonation of a given tone shifts its régister mechanism to the type of the next lower register. This phenomenon is especially noticeable at register transition points. It seems only logical, then, that blending of registers should precede bigness of sound. Particularly in young, developing voices, an even scale should be achieved before attempting the demands of a Verdi aria.

Lehmann, in her usual florid style, calls the head voice (light mechanism) the singer's guardian angel and an indispensible tool in blending registers.[56]

> Without its aid all voices lack brilliancy and carrying power; they are like a head without a brain. Only by constantly summoning it to the aid of all other registers is the singer able to keep this voice fresh and youthful. Only by a

> careful application of it do we gain that power of endurance which enables us to meet the most fatiguing demands. By it alone can we effect a complete equalization of the whole compass of all voices, and extend that compass.

These words of a legendary singer who performed Isolde when she was sixty and sang lieder recitals past the age of 70 certainly cannot be dismissed as idle chatter. Vocal endurance and a seamless scale were the distinguishing characteristics of this voice, a voice that was heard in major opera houses for over fifty years.

Ascending intervals, particularly over a register bridge, often are troublesome. The quality and weight of the higher pitch must be anticipated and prepared for in the lower one. Two of the great singers of this century had words of wisdom about this problem. Enrico Caruso said:

> In the matter of taking high notes one should remember that their purity and ease of production depend very much on the way the preceding notes leading up to them are sung.[57]

The German baritone, Gerhard Huesch, spoke often of "the tone before the tone" and cautioned that it should not be "too rich."[58]

Even in the mid-1980s, questions about vocal registers continue to be asked. There is much that is still under investigation and as yet unexplained. A few singing teachers continue to believe that the "natural" voice has no registers and that the changes of quality heard in most voices are solely the result of faulty technique. Most of their colleagues disagree with that view. The majority of scientists base their belief that registers do exist on well-supported laboratory observations. Whatever one's orientation, all concur that equilization of vocal quality is the hallmark of good singing technique and a key pedagogical goal. In 1909 Luisa Tetrazzini understood the basic components needed to attain this goal.

> This blending of the registers is obtained by the intelligence of the singer in mixing the different tone qualities of the registers, using as aids the various formations of the lips, mouth and throat and the ever present appoggio without which no perfect scale can be sung.[59]

Voice Classification

Voice types usually are divided into bass, baritone, tenor, contralto, mezzo-soprano, and soprano. Subclassifications, such as coloratura, lyric, dramatic, and buffo, depend to a certain extent upon cultural preferences, individual personality or temperament, and suitability of body type for the stage. In recent years, casting has often depended as much on appearance as upon vocal timbre and voice classification.

The measurement of such anatomical features as the length and thickness of vocal folds when at rest, the volume of the resonating tract, and the overall body structure can give some indication of classification. There are many more tall baritones than there are tall tenors. Short, broad vocal folds are typical of tenors and sopranos, while long, narrow cords predominate in basses and contraltos. In general, small resonators are found in high sopranos. All of these tendencies, however, are just that--tendencies only. Many singers have sounds which simply are not in agreement with their physical characteristics. A young baritone with all the physical attributes of his voice type may have the ringing high tones of a tenor. Which is he? How should he be trained?

There are many theories of how to classify a young voice empirically, almost as many as there are singing teachers. The basic components of most of these theories are timbre, tessitura, and range. At the risk of repeating earlier material, definitions will assure mutual understanding of what these terms mean. Timbre or tone color is an amalgam of the fundamental, the number and distribution of its harmonics, and the respective amplitudes of these harmonics. The sound wave which determines timbre is the result of breath management, vocal fold function, and resonator adjustment. Range is the extent of a voice, the upper and lower limits of frequency. Within that range, there is a certain compass in which the voice performs with special ease of production and sound. That compass of notes is called the tessitura.

Probably the least reliable and the most dangerous way to classify a voice is by range. Other than indicating whether a voice is male or female, a relatively simple judgment to make about normal voices, range is a "sometime thing." Particularly in young voices, it can bob up and down like a yo-yo. A mezzo-soprano range is common for a young soprano who has not yet found the light or head voice. Young male singers frequently have the low notes of a bass and may eventually become baritones or even tenors. A conclusive range is almost always a product of vocal maturity and, as such, is of little use as a tool to classify voices during training.

Timbre is undoubtedly a better estimator of classification than range. Since timbre is so closely related to formant frequencies, it should give some indication of the size and dimensions of the vocal tract. At the same time, timbre is determined to a great extent by the particular method of voice training. A young baritone who sings with a very dark color, i.e., emphasis on the lower harmonics, may very well have first formant frequencies of a bass, regardless of what his natural vocal timbre may be. Sundberg believes that the development of a voice timbre in voice training is a matter of learning a special articulation.[60]

Another problem with the use of timbre is its deceiving aural nature. If a young female has a naturally darker singing voice than her peers, she generally is classified as a mezzo. Many a big-voiced soprano has sung as a mezzo into her mid-20's, only to find that her voice was misclassified. The retraining period can be extended and frustrating because the upper third of her voice has been inactive for so long. As a result, sometimes the voice never reaches its full potential. The sad thing about this kind of classification by timbre alone is that the rare voices, such as the spinto soprano and the dramatic tenor, are the ones most often misclassified. At best, their potential is never realized; at worst, permanent vocal damage results.

Tessitura and the careful monitoring of bridges between registers is the most viable way to classify young voices. Classification becomes a tentative rather than a definitive assessment, is always under consideration, and is subject to change when circumstances warrant. The tessitura, that compass of notes to which a particular singer's voice naturally inclines, changes with training and age. Over and over, one reads that great care and caution should be exercised, and that professional voice classification cannot be determined until time and hard work have worked their magic.

The singing voice is considered a young instrument from the time it changes during puberty to the age of 25. Muscular maturation continues during those years. For instance, very few singers develop the extrinsic laryngeal muscles before 21 or 22 years of age. When they do, laryngeal positioning changes both phonatory and resonating capabilities. Fluidity and ease of production are important goals during these formative years, and most singers profit from training as lyrics, regardless of potential. Of course, the big voices take until 30 or even 35 years of age to attain full maturity. How ridiculous then for a young singer to call himself or herself a "dramatic!" At the other extreme, a small voice, no matter how beautiful it may sound in a small room, must be allowed to develop at its own pace. Sometimes it grows in size and sometimes it does not. Attempts to make it bigger than it really is can ruin the quality and cause great disappointment and heartache. Very rarely do slightly-built, short people with narrow chests and small heads and necks become opera singers. For a more detailed description of characteristics of the young voice, see Appendix I.

The matter of voice classification seems to be almost continually on the minds of serious young singers. They ask for a definitive assessment at almost every lesson. Teachers who rely on someone else's impressive but not very valid theory of how to classify voices do a disservice to their students. Instead they need good ears, an assortment of evasive answers, and a strong conviction that all things come to those who wait. A wise answer to "what kind of voice am I?" is "better than you were last week."

Vibrato

Major Characteristics

The presence of vibrato in the singing sound has long been recognized as an important part of the timbre or quality. It has been estimated that vibrato is found in 95% of all "classically" sung tones. Tastes in amplitude and even at times in the speed of the vibrato have varied during different periods in the history of western vocal music, but the consistency or evenness of the vibrato pattern seems to have remained a desirable attribute. The straight tone is heard today primarily in popular vocal styles. Many authorities on Renaissance and pre-Renaissance music also believe that vibratoless singing was used during that period. To ears accustomed to the vibrato in western vocal music of the past three hundred years, the straight tone often sounds slightly below the pitch.

What is vibrato? Because it apparently is the result of a freely functioning total instrument, it defies description except as a perceptual phenomenon, and even such a definition is dependent upon teaching methods and aesthetic preferences. For example, a well-known voice teacher calls vibrato "... impulses which cause the tone to be buoyant, harmonically rich, flexible, and whose oscillating pattern is not perceived as such."[61] When voice scientists participated in a panel on vocal vibrato at the 1986 Symposium on Care of the Professional Voice, their conclusions were almost as subjective. Michel: "It's probably going to be made in a lot of different ways by a lot of different people."[62] Sundberg, although quantifying the phenomenon as a product of subglottic pressure, fundamental frequency, and formant frequencies, was also equivocal.[63]

> I would expect that it would be very difficult to find any systematic changes, or even any of the means for the singer to vary this amplitude vibrato systematically.

Dr. Van Lawrence, in his usual candid manner, spoke of the variation in vibratos seen in premier singers at Houston Opera.[64]

> ... I have seen over the years very little similar vibrato appearance in any of my premier singers. This was a very astounding thing, too, at first. I thought that everyone would produce vibrato in the same way and thereby give me the same laryngeal picture. But this is not so. I have seen some vibrato that I am aware of acoustically and this is not visible by any movement on the television monitor screen. ...So in my book, the vibrato production will be very different from one singer to the other.

Thus even in all the measurable parameters, a great variety of results occurs, and certain acoustical perceptions are not visible at all in the larynx.

To the ears of the average listener, a fluid vibrato is not heard as such, but is perceived as an integral part of the timbre. From an acoustical point of view, however, the "beats" of a vibrato define the musical texture of a tone. They add harmonic richness and give the impression that a tone is centered on pitch. Put another way, Benade says that a "fair amount of vibrato ... adds a great deal of recognizability to the various sinusoidal components of the voice by providing them with a synchronized pulsation in frequency and amplitude (as they sweep across their various formants)."[65] This increased recognizability in the presence of vibrato may be the reason for the inadequate auditory recognition of some straight tones. In the singing of many children and in that of early music performers, the sound is literally pure; it has very few harmonics, and the vibrato is extremely narrow in its oscillation from the mean frequency. Again, however, cultural preference is a determinant because children in some countries (Austria) sing with vibrato while those in other countries (England) do not.

There are three main parameters in the phenomenon of vibrato. These elements were reported by Carl Seashore and his research team at the University of Iowa in the 1930's. Countless investigators since then have verified these findings.

(1) number per second of the oscillations
(2) variation in intensity (amplitude)
(3) fluctuation of pitch

It is generally agreed that five to seven oscillations per second are found in well trained singing voices, although the oscillation rate decreases in soft singing and becomes more pronounced with growing vocal intensity, according to Winckel (1953).[66] The vibrato rate for men is often slower than for women. Seldom does a male vibrato reach the rate of seven per second.

During each oscillation there is an intensity change of from two decibels to as much as eight decibels. The lower figure is more common. There is, however, no difference between men and women in the degree of intensity (amplitude) possible at a given pitch level.[67]

Pitch fluctuation around a mean frequency can be as great as a semitone, or a quartertone on either side of the mean. Again, there is no difference between men and women in the extent of these fluctuations.

A vibrato with a low number of oscillations (three to four per second) is frequently found among singers of popular music. Most concert and opera singers of high repute have a vibrato with five to six oscillations per second and fluctuations of about a semitone.

Among classical singers, a vibrato which is irregular and rapid in rate (more than seven times per second) and which has wide fluctuations in pitch and in intensity is called a tremolo. If a low number of oscillations per second is accompanied by wide fluctuations of pitch, the result is called a wobble. Such a condition can be caused by age, by muscle fatigue, or by an overly weighty, dark production. Despite the fact that scientists have no data on the causes of either tremolo or wobble (they are still working on causes of the normal vibrato!), Vennard thinks that certain exaggerations of the normal vibrato, the tremolo in particular, are sometimes caused by muscle "overloading."[68] Muscular coordination is out of balance; the breath stream is not hooking up smoothly with laryngeal function. If a muscle is overtaxed, a tremor occurs, and the greater the overload on that muscle, the greater the trembling. All of us have seen trembling tongues, jaws, and even entire larynxes, during the singing act. All are signs of excessive tension.

From a teaching point of view, it is not helpful to badger students about tremolos. They only become more nervous and try to control the sound. This kind of vocal problem is as much an emotional and psychological one as it is physical. A positive pedagogical approach is more likely to encourage self-confidence and relaxation than continual prodding and admonishing.

The Trill

With the increase in interest in and knowledge about the performance practice of the Renaissance and Baroque periods, it is advantageous for a singer to know how to trill.

Unlike the vibrato, the trill is initiated voluntarily and is specifically measured musically with a rapid alternation at a major or minor second, depending upon its position in the scale. Garcia said it is produced "by a very loose and swift oscillation of the larynx."[69] When asked whether the trill is related to the vibrato, all seven panelists at the Care of the Professional Voice Symposium (1979) said no.[70] All are research scientists. When asked how to teach a person to trill, however, there was only the comment that "there is still a great deal to be learned about trill production."[71]

Although it is begun and ended deliberately, generally at a comparatively slow tempo, the concentration necessary to keep a long trill within bounds plus the abandon needed to allow it to really establish itself are very difficult to achieve for many singers. If Garcia is right and the entire larynx moves, then looseness and freedom of movement probably should precede any intellectual measurement of rhythmic divisions, at least for a singer who is trying to develop the skill. Many teachers, on the other hand, use measured exercises at a definite tempo which is then doubled and redoubled until finally the trill emerges. Vennard tells of a student who sang a slow trill and then was asked to "throw in the flutter as if giggling or chuckling." She said it felt like "a very loose note."[72]

Causes of Vibrato

The desirability of a fluid, even vibrato is not in doubt. What causes this phenomenon is.

The acoustic characteristics of the vibrato in singing have been extensively documented, but there is comparatively little indisputable evidence about its physiological causes. From Seashore to current research projects, a multitude of studies and educated guesses have been put forth. Most of the reports deal with specific activities, such as abdominal/diaphragmatic effort, crico-thyroid activity, and subglottic air pressure. In 1966, Mason and Zemlin, using surface electrodes, found that the crico-thyroid pulsates in synchronization with the pitch and intensity fluctuations of the vibrato.[73] No other intrinsic laryngeal muscle is that closely related to vibrato. Appelman maintains that the cause of vibrato is controlled undulations of the diaphragm.[74] In 1979, Large reported that "the physiological control of vocal vibrato is combined laryngeal and respiratory mechanism, with the laryngeal factor predominating."[75]

There is no doubt that a legato line is possible only with a steady breath flow and a fluid, even vibrato. How to achieve either (or both) is argued vehemently, and the jury is still out. Thus far no one has studied the effect of resonance tract adjustments on vibrato, although the quantification of the acoustic properties of vibrato represents the great majority of studies done on the phenomenon.

Because attributing the physical cause of vibrato to a localized and limited part of the singing mechanism has provided only a partial explanation, a more global approach may be necessary. Is it a result of nerve impulses? Maybe. In addition to singing sounds, it is found in normal speech, laughter, and bird and insect calls. Personal temperament and emotional state at a specific time are things which all voice teachers must cope with continually. In addition to these complex elements, consider how often vibrato is altered to fulfill musical demands. It is an integral part of expressiveness, and as such is subconsciously modified when appropriate.

Vibrato, then, is a multi-factorial process. Some teachers feel that it should never be taught because it appears as the result of proper coordinaton and efficiency of function. They teach the technique by which vibrato is attained. Others believe that vibrato can be taught directly, and they do so. Controversy is raging as strongly among singing teachers as among their colleagues in the research laboratories.

A fluid and even vibrato is certainly an indication that things are going right, just as an irregular vibrato pattern is a sign of trouble. Vennard thinks that an uneven vibrato "... can be cured, not by a few tricks, but by gradually learning the correct technique. When the singer is producing as he should, he will have a normal vibrato."[76] Coffin says that an irregular vibrato is a sign that "there is a fight going on between vocal cord vibration, vocal tract resonation, and the breath."[77] On the basis of aural perception, visual observation, and what laboratory evidence there is, it seems probable that a regular, free-flowing vibrato is the result of the intricate functional interdependence of the total singing instrument.

NOTES

1. James McKinney, *The Diagnosis and Correction of Vocal Faults* (Nashville, TN : Broadman Press, 1982), 97.

2. Garcia, *Hints*, op. cit., 8.

3. Raymond H. Colton, "Physiological Mechanisms of Vocal Frequency Control: The Role of Tension," *Journal of Voice*, 2:3 (1988), 208.

4. Vennard, *Singing*, op. cit., 86.

5. Carol Schoenhard and Harry Hollien, "A Perceptual Study of Registration in Female Singers," *NATS Bulletin*, 39:1 (1982), 23.

6. Lehmann, op. cit., 111.

7. MacKenzie, op. cit., 45.

8. Shakespeare, op. cit., 21.

9. Hollien, Harry, "Review of Vocal Registers," *Care of the Professional Voice*, Transcripts of the Twelfth Symposium, Part I, Van Lawrence, ed. New York: Voice Foundation, 1983, 5 (the list of registers was a consensus of common vocal registers made by the Collegium Medicorum Theatre, a society consisting primarily of physicians).

10. Ibid.

11. Vennard, *Singing*, op. cit., 69-73.

12. Stan Hill, "Characteristics of Air Flow During Changes in Registration," *NATS Journal*, 43:1 (1986), 17.

13. Craig Timberlake, "Terminological Turmoil: The Naming of Registers," *NATS Journal*, 47:1 (1990), 25.

14. Thomas Shipp, Robert Coleman, John Large, Charles Beard, Cynthia Hoffman, Daniel Pratt, and Ingo Titze [panel], "Have We Learned Anything About Registers?", *Care of the Professional Voice*, Transcripts of the 9th Symposium, Part I, Van Lawrence, ed. (New York: Voice Foundation, 1980), 126.

15. Ibid.

16. Ingo R. Titze, "Vocal Registers," *NATS Bulletin*, 39:4 (1983), 22.

17. Paul B. Oncley, "Dual Concept of Singing Registers," *Vocal Registers in Singing*, John Large, ed. (The Hague: Mouton, 1973), 43.

18. Godfrey E. Arnold, "Research Potentials in Voice Registers," *Vocal Registers*, John Large, ed., Ibid., 138.

19. Large and Murray, op. cit., 14.

20. Mathilde Marchesi, *Theoretical and Practical Vocal Method*. Reprint (New York: Dover, 1970), xv.

21. Vennard, *Singing*, op. cit., 76.

22. Marchesi, op. cit., xv.

23. Garcia, *Hints*, op. cit., 9-10.

24. Ibid., 15.

25. Brodnitz, op. cit., 63. The book is dedicated to Manuel Garcia.

26. William Earl Brown, *Vocal Wisdom* (New York: Arno Press, 1931), 137.

27. Garcia, *Hints*, op. cit., 7.

28. Arnold Rose, *The Singer and the Voice* (London: Faber and Faber, 1962), 148.

29. Garcia, *Hints*, op. cit., 9.

30. Statement by Marilyn Horne, quoted in Coffin, *Sounds*, op. cit., 113.

31. Henry Pleasants, *The Great Singers* (New York: Simon and Schuster, 1966), 272.

32. Zemlin, *Speech and Hearing*, op. cit., 166.

33. Hollien, *Review of Vocal Registers*, op. cit., 5.

34. Ibid.

35. Personal conversation in July, 1980.

36. Garcia, *Hints*, op. cit., 17.

37. William Vennard and Minoru Hirano, "Varieties of Voice Production," *NATS Bulletin*, 27:3 (1971), 26-32.

38. Stella Hertegard, Jan Gauffin, and Johan Sundberg, "Open and Covered Singing as Studied by Means of Fiberoptics, Inverse Filtering, and Spectral Analysis," *Journal of Voice*, 4:3 (1990), 220-230.

39. Vennard and Hirano, "Varieties," op. cit., 28.

40. Minoru Hirano, Lecture at *The Biology of Music Making*, Denver, Colorado, July 10, 1984.

41. Vennard, *Singing*, op. cit., 68.

42. Hirano, Denver lecture, op. cit., (1984).

43. Yoshiyuki Horii, "Jitter and Shimmer in Sustained Vocal Fry Phonation," *Folia Phoniatrica*, 37 (1985), 81-86.

44. M. C. Ametrano Jackson, "The High Male Range," *Folia Phoniatrica*, 39 (1987), 20.

45. Robert Thayer Sataloff, Barry C. Baron, Friedrich S. Brodnitz, Van L. Lawrence, Wallace Rubin, Joseph Spiegel, and Gayle Woodson [panel], "Acute Medical Problems of the Voice," *Journal of Voice*, 2:4 (1988), 352.

46. Ibid.

47. Van Lawrence, "Laryngological Observations on Belting," *Journal of Research in Singing*, 2:1 (1979), 26-28.

48. Robert Edwin, "To Belt or Not to Belt--Maybe Is the Answer," *NATS Journal*, 44:3 (1988), 39.

49. Jo Estill, "Observations about the Quality Called 'Belting'," Transcripts of the Ninth Symposium; *Care of the Professional Voice*, Part 2, Van Lawrence, ed. (New York: The Voice Foundation, 1980), 82-88.

50. Jo Estill, "Belting and Classic Voice Quality: Some Physiological Differences," *Medical Problems of Performing Artists*, 3:1 (1988), 42.

51. Ibid., 38.

52. Beth Miles and Harry Hollien, "Whither Belting," *Journal of Voice*, 4:1 (1990), 69.

53. Jan Sullivan, "How to Teach the Belt/Pop Voice," *Journal of Research in Singing*, 13:1 (1989), 44.

54. Miles & Hollien, op. cit., 66.

55. Edwin, op. cit., 39-40.

56. Lehmann, op. cit., 89.

57. Caruso and Tetrazzini, op. cit., 55.

58. From coaching sessions at the University of Colorado, 1978-1979.

59. Caruso and Tetrazzini, op. cit., 28.

60. Johan Sundberg, "The Source Spectrum in Professional Singing," *Folia Phoniatrica*, 25:3 (1973), 87.

61. Cornelius L. Reid, "The Nature of Vibrato," *Journal of Research in Singing*, 12:2 (1989), 44.

62. Robert F. Coleman, Jean Hakes, Douglas M. Hicks, John F. Michel, Lorraine A. Ramig, Howard B. Rothman [panel], "Discussion on Vibrato," *Journal of Voice*, 1:2 (1987), 168.

63. Ibid., 169.

64. Ibid.

65. Benade, op. cit., 381.

66. Cited in Luchsinger and Arnold, op. cit., 93.

67. Thomas Shipp, Rolf Leanderson, and Johan Sundberg, "Rate and Extent of Vibrato as a Function of Vowel, Effort and Frequency," *Care of the Professional Voice*, Transcripts of the 8th Symposium, Part I (New York: Voice Foundation, 1979), 47.

68. Vennard, *Singing*, op. cit., 194-195.

69. Garcia, *Hints*, op. cit., 42.

70. Harry Hollien, Kenneth Neilson, Howard Rothman, K. Izdebski, William Campbell, Thomas Shipp, John Large, Robert Coleman [Panel], "Physical Factors in Voice/Vocal Vibrato," *Care of the Professional Voice*, transcripts of the Eighth

Symposium, Part I, Van Lawrence and Bernd Weinberg, eds. (1980), 64.

71. Ibid.

72. Vennard, *Singing*, op. cit., 203.

73. Robert M. Mason and Willard R. Zemlin, "The Phenomenon of Vocal Vibrato," *NATS Bulletin*, 22:3 (1966), 37.

74. Appelman, *The Science*, op. cit., 23-24, and the 8th (1979) and 14th Symposium (1985) on *Care of the Professional Voice.*

75. John Large, "An Air Flow Study of Vocal Vibrato," *Care of the Professional Voice*, transcripts of the Eighth Symposium, Part I, Van Lawrence and Bernd Weinberg, eds. (New York: Voice Foundation, 1979), 44.

76. Vennard, *Singing*, op. cit., 194.

77. Coffin, *Overtones*, op. cit., 14.

Chapter 9

THE FUNCTIONAL UNITY OF THE SINGING VOICE: A GESTALT

Webster's dictionary defines *gestalt* as a structure of physical phenomena so integrated as to constitute a functional unit. The layman's understanding of gestalt is that the whole is greater than the sum of its parts. The singing mechanism is a perfect example of a gestalt since it can function correctly only when all of its components are working together. Although we have dealt in some detail with specific anatomical parts of the singing mechanism, the study of these parts is an artificial separation for the purpose of instructional clarity. The three major functions of respiration, phonation, and resonation are actually an inseparable unit, and when this unit is operating properly, a cyclical interplay takes place. Weakness or excessive tension in individual muscles will throw the entire system out of balance. Instead, every muscle must maintain whatever tension or relaxation is needed at any given time for the desired sound. Learning how to achieve this equilibrium with a minimum of effort is the principal goal of training.

Of course, functional freedom in singing is not solely a matter of muscle behavior or even of superior breathing techniques. Like the chicken and the egg, one cannot say that these factors are more essential than optimum resonation or vice versa because they are interdependent functions. There is reason to believe, nevertheless, that unless resonance factors are understood, all other training will be for naught. G. B. Lamperti (1839-1910), the teacher of Marcella Sembrich and other famous 19th century singers, says that "it is a strange fact that the throat is controlled by what happens above it, in the acoustics of the head, through word, vibration and resonance."[1] In a 1988 study, Rothenberg reports that "... singers may be expected to vary in the degree to which they employ tuning to create pressure-flow phase relationships at the glottis that maximize the oscillatory energy in the vocal folds. ..."[2] Marvin W. Luttges, a physicist, believes that "laryngeal vibration is relatively crude and sloppy. The main task of a good singer is to shape his sound filters to enhance the desired sound."[3] Thus distuning of the resonators produces a corresponding imbalance in the release of air and in vocal fold vibration.

On the other hand, easy emission of sound depends on the mastery of adequate breath energy, the motor of the voice. Subglottic air pressure is determined by the coordination and voluntary control of respiratory activity. The resulting balance of forces has a major effect upon efficient use of air by the glottal lips. An unsteady, fluctuating air stream or one which is held back has a negative effect upon vocal fold vibration and the ensuing sound wave. The resonators consequently cannot adequately amplify a deficient sound spectrum.

In either case, that of resonance distuning or of inefficient breathing techniques, undesirable tension occurs.

Consider two examples of vocal dysfunction caused by excessive muscular tension. If too much intensity and/or too much weight is used in the middle voice, excessive medial compression of the vocal folds is used, thereby overworking the lateral crico-arytenoids and underworking the inter-arytenoids. Such muscular imbalance causes vocal fold dysfunction and possible physical damage. Clavicular breathing produces tension in the collarbone and neck areas and makes muscular equilibrium of the extrinsic network difficult or even impossible. Then the larynx rides too high, and efficient phonation and resonation are impaired.

We mentioned earlier the adverse effect upon the vocal folds when the resonating tube is not appropriately shaped. Those singers who discount the acoustical laws concerning vowel formants and the need for vowel modification will attain a free, fluid sound only with great difficulty. They also are likely to develop debilitating tensions in the tongue, jaw, or soft palate. Poorly tuned resonators and the resulting tension in the articulators will also cause inefficient use of the breath.

Mathilde Marchesi understood the primary importance of mastery of the craft of singing.

> Every art consists of a technical-mechanical part and an aesthetical part. A singer who cannot overcome the difficulties of the first part can never attain perfection in the second, not even a genius.[4]

When the voice works as a functional unit, it allows singers to develop an extended range with an even scale, a seamless legato, secure intonation regardless of vowel, tessitura, and dynamic, sufficient transmission or projection of sound, and a wide palette of colors. These are the sensuous building blocks of their art. With these basic components, mastery of that art is possible. Without them, it is not. Ultimately, to achieve the gestalt or functional unity of the singing voice is the goal of all singers.

NOTES

1. Brown, op. cit., 66.

2. Martin Rothenberg, "Acoustic Reinforcement of Vocal Fold Vibratory Behavior in Singing," Chapter 34, *Vocal Physiology: Voice Production, Mechanisms and Functions*, Osamu Fujimura, ed. (New York: Raven Press, 1988), 386.

3. Marvin W. Luttges, Professor of Physics, University of Colorado at Boulder, from a lecture delivered October 4, 1977.

4. Marchesi, op. cit., xviii.

Appendix I

VOCAL ABUSE AND MISUSE

What is a hoarse sound? A husky voice? A breathy tone? Because aural perception is such a subjective matter and there is no standard by which to measure a tone, there is no common vocabulary to describe what we hear. To further complicate the problem, those professionals directly concerned with the condition and behavior of the larynx approach the subject from entirely different perspectives. The laryngologist is a medical doctor who diagnoses the physiological behavior underlying a vocal disorder. The voice scientist is generally an M.D. or a Ph. D. who has the objective perspective of a research scientist. The voice therapist works to correct organic or functional problems and return the voice to a normal state. The singing teacher, using intangible criteria dictated by his/her hearing and training, seeks a tone quality appropriate for a particular singing voice. Naturally enough, communication between these disciplines is not easy. It is essential, then, that singing teachers learn as much as possible about all three of these allied fields.

It is extremely helpful for the singing teacher to form a professional working relationship with a trusted and understanding laryngologist. Not all laryngologists seem to understand the singer's temperament and the unique physical demands of singing. Those who do are often self-educated about singers, have had extensive private practice experience, or consult frequently with knowledgeable voice teachers and voice therapists. You have found a gem if he or she understands the impact of certain voice techniques on vocal production. For example, if a laryngologist finds that the lateral crico-arytenoids are overworking and the inter-arytenoids are underworking so that there is a chink between the arytenoid cartilages, it is indeed unusual to have him/her ask whether the singer is using an unusually dark, heavy production in the middle voice. Yet that is exactly what happened with a mezzo-soprano who recently returned to the United States after several years of study in Germany. In any event, do not hesitate to send a student to a laryngologist as soon as anything atypical is heard. Do not be concerned about frightening the student because the alternative, malfunctioning vocal folds, is worse. If you cannot find someone who has had a lot of experience with singers, look for a young laryngologist who is eager to increase his/her understanding of the singing voice.

A written report from the laryngologist outlining the nature and the severity of a singer's condition is an invaluable aid to the singing teacher. Then if there is any unfamiliar terminology or the teacher has further questions, there is a basis on which to confer. This kind of written record also is helpful when talking to the student, particularly if the problem is not severe or is an imaginary one. Reassurance from an M.D. is worth a thousand words from the teacher. Unfortunately, a great many voice teachers are not comfortable with this kind of collaborative relationship because they do not know enough about the physical nature of the larynx. If that is the case, it would be wise to learn how that amazing little box works. After all, one does not actually have to become a doctor, but only to understand enough about laryngeal anatomy to talk knowledgeably **with** a doctor. If, on the other hand, the singing teacher resents what is considered interference on the part of the laryngologist, and the latter neither knows nor understands the specific problems of singing, the student is the one who suffers. The resulting damage can be irreparable.

If a student has a functional imbalance which seems to warrant the services of a voice therapist, the same kind of professional trust and communication is needed. Some voice therapists are trained to work exclusively with the speaking voice and have only a vague understanding of the sustained air stream, the greatly expanded frequency range, and the significance of vowel formants to the singing voice. Consequently, it is crucial to find a therapist who does recognize the differences.

There's something in my throat!

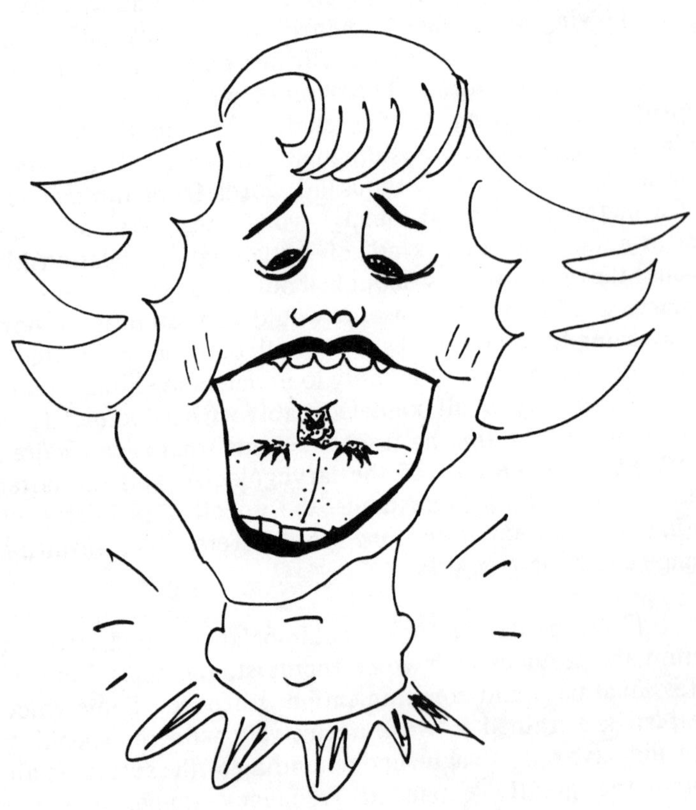

Physical Disorders

Whereas vocal abuse is the mistreatment of the vocal folds, vocal misuse is incorrect use of (1) pitch, (2) volume, (3) breath support, (4) resonance balance, or (5) any combination of these elements. It is extremely difficult, if not impossible, however, to separate organic problems from functional ones. For example, continuous abuse of the vocal folds can lead to nodules, and thus the organic disorder is a direct result of functional misuse. Indeed, almost all vocal damage takes place in the larynx, generally caused by either over-adduction or under-adduction of the vocal folds. The interrelationship of breathing, phonation, and resonation factors in singing makes the cause-and-effect chain a complex gestalt. Contrary to normal expectations, too much muscular force in the breathing process may produce under-adduction of sections of the cords, while lack of muscular equilibrium in the extrinsic musculature generally results in over-adduction of the cords. The result is not always predictable, but it is certain that muscular imbalance is inefficient, even if it does not always result in perceptible physical damage.

It cannot be too strongly stated that vocal abuse, particularly the muscular imbalance resulting from the use of excessive force, does not always produce immediately discernible vocal problems or organic disorders. It may be months or even years before the damage caused by continual abusive habits is evidenced in a pathology such as vocal nodes. Unfortunately, this kind of cumulative damage often is irreversible; the vocal instrument has been injured permanently.

The admonition to "sing on your interest, not your principal" describes a singer who avoids undue tension. This kind of singing achieves a maximum of tonal effect with a minimum of effort. Physical action that is smooth and efficient, relying on neither hyperfunction (over) or hypofunction (under) is not easy to acquire or to maintain in today's world. "Tenseness of muscle groups is a common occurrence in modern civilization. We live in a tense age, and ... vocal hyperfunction belongs to the large number of psychosomatic disorders that translate inner tension into tense organic behavior."[1]

Vocal Nodules and Vocal Polyps

Physical Characteristics

No vocal disorder generates greater fear in the hearts of trained singers than vocal nodes. Sometimes called the corns of the vocal folds, these thick bumps prevent the cords from meeting completely and lead to a raspy, breathy production and a lower fundamental frequency for speakers. For singers, perceptual evidence of nodules includes:

(1) a breathy middle register
(2) "cracking" when approaching the head register
(3) reduction in amount of phonatory time possible
(4) reduction in intensity range
(5) hoarseness

Since nodules are generally bilateral (on both sides), there is obvious chinking of that section of the glottis. An accompanying symptom is a need to clear the throat constantly as if to remove some obstruction on the folds.

Fortunately, many classical singers or their teachers detect the presence of nodules in their early stages when they can be treated relatively easily with vocal therapy or with a change in the kind of literature being sung. A somewhat veiled timbre at lower dynamic levels, a slight "buzz" at the beginning of phonation, and instability in the passaggio are common indications that a laryngeal examination is in order. Certainly the presence of any or even all of these signs does not necessarily mean that nodules are present. "Many singers develop bilateral, symmetrical, soft swellings at the junction of the anterior and middle thirds of their vocal cords after heavy use. There is no evidence to suggest that singers with such 'physiologic swelling' are predisposed toward developing vocal nodes."[2] Sataloff goes on to say that this kind of swelling generally disappears after 48 hours of rest from heavy voice use.

Before discussing the probable causes of this condition, a more detailed picture of vocal fold structure is needed. According to Hirano,[3] the vocal cords have three outer mucosal layers covered by a thin membranous tissue or epithelium. Underneath the thin membrane covering the vocal folds is the lamina propria comprised of three mucosal layers. The first layer, called Reinke's space, resembles a mass of soft gelatin, and is very pliable. The second layer consists of elastic fibers with the consistency of soft rubber bands. The deepest layer is made up primarily of collagenous fibers like cotton thread. These last two layers together are called the vocal ligament. Below that is the vocalis muscle, the main body of the vocal folds; it is like a bundle of stiff rubber bands. The more superficial the layer, the more pliable it is. From a mechanical point of view, Hirano says that these layers can be divided into three sections.[4]

(1) the cover or epithelium and Reinke's space
(2) the transition layer consisting of the intermediate and deep layers of the lamina propria (also designated the vocal ligament)
(3) the vocalis muscle

Although these three structures have many connective tissues and appear to move as one unit during vibration, Hirano believes that the epithelium and the first layer actually move in a different manner from the remaining layers.[5] At any rate, it is well established that tissue reactions to vocal stress almost always take place in the first mucosal layer, Reinke's Space. It is there, in the superficial or outer layer of the folds, that vocal nodes form; they generally do not extend into the vocal ligament.[6] The total diameter of the epithelium plus Reinke's Space is only about 1.1 millimeters, so a vocal nodule is very small, but then, comparatively speaking, so are the vocal folds themselves.

Dr. Robert J. Feder, one of the most highly regarded laryngeal surgeons in the country, says that most vocal nodules do not need to be surgically removed.[7] The majority of them can be treated successfully with a carefully monitored program of voice therapy. If surgery does need to be performed, however, Dr. Feder says that every effort should be made to preserve the vocal ligament. In other words, if the elastic tissue just below Reinke's Space is not violated and the vocal ligament is not entered, minimal scarring will take place. Post-operative voice therapy can then be done much more successfully since scarring disrupts normal mucosal vibration. The traditional practice of "stripping" the cords during nodular surgery is an outdated procedure that should be relegated to the medical trashcan.

The sound produced by vocal polyps is similar to that of nodules, hoarse, breathy, and rough. Their physical characteristics are somewhat different, however. Most polyps are the result of vocal fold hemorrhaging which, when absorbed, leaves the tissue swollen and distended. Whereas the vocal nodule is a callous formation, the polyp generally has the structure of a small, engorged blood vessel.[8] Some polyps are broad based and sit on the edge of the vocal fold, while others are attached to the fold by a narrow neck. The latter sometimes hang below the adducted vocal cords, and because they do not interfere with cordal vibration, no voice changes are heard. Polyps sometimes are as large as cherry stones, but unlike nodules, they are more likely to be unilateral (on one side only) rather than bilateral.

Typically, both nodules and polyps appear at the junction of the anterior and middle third of the cord, at what is actually the midpoint of the membranous portion of the vibrating cord. Polyps, unlike vocal nodules, are frequently caused by a single traumatic event such as continuous yelling at a sporting event.

Causes

Abuse of the voice is the major cause of vocal nodes. If there is excessive tensing of the vocal folds and excessive force in their adduction, nodes may appear, and once they have formed, they disturb vocal cord closure and vibration, creating additional damage. The two major functional causes of nodes are using breath pressure that is too high and/or using glottal attacks. The fact that nodes are most common in sopranos and tenors[9] substantiates such a diagnosis. Singers of both classifications sometimes try to produce high notes with sufficient volume by the chronic use of glottal attacks. If the young singer (under 30) sings at an extremely high tessitura, particularly too loudly and for too long a time, he/she risks permanent damage. When the "bloom" of a voice is destroyed, it almost never comes back.

> ... we know what mad things a young singer will do to play a coveted part--with the connivance of a manager at his wit's end to find voices that can encompass popular operatic parts at salaries that will not bankrupt the company.[10]

Since vocal nodules interfere with the proper thinning and stiffening of the cords, they cause particular difficulty in singing high notes, and singing softly is almost impossible. As the cords are forced together more and more violently to "get" the note, the physical problem increases. Singers who belt (and their speaking counterparts, cheerleaders) use very high breath pressure **plus** the glottal attack, and they use these abusive behaviors for unusually long periods of time. No wonder the incidence of vocal nodes is so high in both groups.

Another kind of vocal production needs to be mentioned here. Among proponents of some German methodologies, a dark sound at high dynamic levels is preferred. Unusually high breath pressure is a characteristic of this method, as is a "tucked-chin" position of the head and neck. Both put excessive tension on the intrinsic and extrinsic muscles of the larynx. In addition, the vowels are "equalized" by maintaining a fairly open and rounded mouth position, a large pharyngeal space, and a depressed larynx. Under these conditions, the lower partials are emphasized and there is a loss of upper partials. More importantly, it is difficult to believe that the physical laws of vowel formants can be implemented when cavity coupling is under such rigid and artificial control.

The extent of undue muscular tension and its effect on the vocal folds is dependent, of course, upon the specific methodology and the individual singer, but if carried to extremes, the method is potentially dangerous. It should be mentioned here that not all German teachers endorse this method. All young singers need to be aware of its dangers, however, and guard against the persuasive teacher who wants to "develop" a bigger and darker voice than is warranted.

If there is too much median pull or muscle mass at middle voice frequencies, the vocalis is overcontracting in order to maintain enough amplitude of vibration, and the lateral crico-arytenoid adductor is overworking in order to keep the cords firmly adducted. In addition to too much tension in the area where vocal nodes usually appear, the local cooling system is being impeded as well because the added friction is creating greater heat and viscosity in the vocal folds. This kind of condition is usually brought about by too much weight and/or too much intensity in the middle voice, particularly in the female singing voice. The middle register in women is an especially troublesome area in which to get enough "focus." Singing louder and heavier is no substitute because it merely throws the voice out of balance. This tendency to abuse and overwork the middle register may be one reason why female singers are more subject to vocal nodes than male singers.

Contact Ulcers

Physical Characteristics

At the posterior end of the vocal folds, the superficial layer of elastic fibers becomes thinner and acts as a shock absorber to protect the ends of the folds from possible mechanical damage caused by vibration.[11] This thin layer attaches to the vocal process of the arytenoid cartilage which is covered with a mucous membrane. An injury to the tissue is called a contact ulcer or granuloma and is usually bilateral, though not always. What is at first an ulcerous lesion may later become grainy or fibrous tissue around the ulcer crater. Primary symptoms are a voice which tires easily, occasional laryngeal pain, and severe inflammation of the vocal processes. Although vocal rest often brings about recovery and an apparent loss of symptoms, they recur more frequently and more severely with the passage of time if the problem which caused the condition is not corrected.

Causes

Obviously, the forceful meeting of the vocal processes, what is more commonly called the hard glottal attack, is the major cause of contact ulcers. As mentioned in the section on vocal nodes, this method of phonation is found in certain singing styles, most notably in "hard rock" and in female singers who belt in a functionally abusive and inefficient way. Some opera singers also use an inordinate number of glottal attacks at very high intensity levels.

People who use unusually low-pitched speaking voices also are subject to contact ulcers. The voice of authority (pastors, army sargeants, lawyers) is generally low-pitched and filled with glottal attacks. Many middle-aged men fit this category. Indeed, contact ulcers are found primarily in men. The hard-driving compulsive perfectionist personality also is particularly subject to this disorder. In the case of both kinds of temperaments, the physical problem seems to have an underlying cause which is at least partially psychosomatic. Although the preferred treatment is vocal rehabilitation, contact ulcers are difficult to treat because the entire concept of self is involved.

Rock singers, with their driving, hypnotic style, are not easily weaned from vocal habits that are so emotionally fulfilling. Although great performers are excitable, volatile people and no audience wants to listen to phlegmatic, placid singers, there is a physical limit to how much stress the vocal folds can endure. Continuous phonation at decibel levels above the pain threshold is not only hurtful to the ears, but also risks the permanent impairment of the vocal mechanism. A recent study (1990) of 57 people with contact ulcers did not agree with the "typical" profile of excessive loudness. Half of the subjects were in relatively low stress jobs and less than half spoke too low.[12] A definitive demographic profile awaits further research.

Other causes of contact ulcers are (1) intubation during general anesthetic surgery and (2) gastroesophageal reflux. The latter condition is especially prevalent among professional singers who often eat and drink late at night after a performance. The best antidote, of course, is several hours between the last meal and going to bed. If the problem persists, raising the head, neck, and torso with a triangular pillow may prevent the wash of acid over the pads of the arytenoids. Avoidance of milk products, caffeine, alcohol, and spicy foods also is recommended.

Endotracheal Intubation

Laryngeal injury occurs to some extent in 100% of all endotracheal intubations.[13] Intubation is the placing of a tube into a hollow organ, such as the trachea, to keep it open. During any surgical procedure in which general anesthesia is administered, a breathing tube is inserted between the vocal folds and into the trachea. At the very least, this foreign body creates undue pressure against the tissue with which it comes in contact, and in many cases irritates the mucous membrane covering the cartilaginous vocal process. Naturally, the longer the pressure is continued, the greater the irritation. Since the tube is removed only after the patient is conscious, though, the period of greatest danger occurs in the recovery room. Head and neck movements and coughing in an attempt to expel the obstruction are followed by drawing the tube out through already-irritated vocal folds.

Despite this grim picture, the percentage of patients who suffer serious injury is very small. Most patients experience some degree of hoarseness or soreness (tenderness) for three days or less, although in some cases the effects can be felt for as much as a month. If symptoms are felt beyond three months, however, a thorough laryngeal examination is indicated.

Because singers are so aware of even minor disturbances in voice production, many talk with their anesthetists before surgery and request more careful treatment, including the use of a pediatric or smaller endotracheal tube. There is no guarantee, however, that the nurses in the recovery room will have received the message. Some cautious singers put a sign reading "singer" on their foreheads.

For the professional voice user, the period following surgery should be supervised by a laryngologist. Generally, a month is needed before full vocal activity can be resumed, but sometimes it takes longer to recover. Like all other athletes, if a minor trauma is not allowed to heal properly, long-term complications can be expected.

Hormonal Changes

The Thyroid Gland

Although too large a subject to treat in detail here, there are certain hormonal changes of specific importance to singers.

The thyroid gland, which produces a hormone that affects metabolic rate, lies at the base of the neck. Hypofunction of this gland lowers vocal pitch and often causes a somewhat coarse sound. The condition is reversible and generally can be treated with medication. If surgery is necessary, however, great care must be taken not to damage the extrinsic muscles of the larynx or the recurrent laryngeal nerve, which lie right next to the thyroid gland.

Menstruation

During the past twenty-five years, scientists have argued about whether or not menstruation affects the singing voice. Based on acoustic and physiological changes reported in numerous studies done in the 1960's and 1970's, most major European opera houses have what are called "respect days." Female singers are not asked to perform during the time immediately prior to and on the first days of menstruation. In contrast, professional female singers in the United States continue to sing during that time. In a 1989 study of 38 women, over 50% showed hoarseness and an increase in vocal fatigue during this period of distinct hormonal changes.[14]

Even granted that there are major individual differences in the degree of hormonal change among women, certain vascular changes definitely do take place. As the estrogen level declines during the premenstrual period, laryngeal tissue begins to absorb water, causing the folds to swell. At the same time, there is an increase in the blood supply to the vocal folds because of greater thyroid gland activity. Increased water and blood supply means the folds have greater mass.

Possible changes in phonation include hoarseness, breathiness, and reduction in range, particularly in the top voice. Although certain recent studies show no significant correlation between these symptoms and the menstrual cycle, other authorities disagree, primarily because these studies use speaking rather than singing voices or data collected from untrained female singers. The substantial demands placed upon the singing voices of professional artists can in no way be equated with either of these two groups. Despite lack of conclusive scientific evidence, anecdotal reports from a substantial majority of female singers indicate that vocal fold condition at the onset of menstruation interferes with normal, freely functioning phonation.

The Male Hormone

The use of any hormone which is related to testosterone, the male sex hormone, causes changes in vocal fold structure in the form of increases in mass similar to those seen during male puberty. If this hormone is taken over a long period of time, the effect sometimes is irreversible. The cords thicken and become uneven, and the connective tissues of the vocal ligaments are altered so that blending registers becomes more difficult.

The androgen structurally related to the male hormone (market name: Danocrine) is frequently used to treat benign fibrocystic breast disease, a very common condition. It is estimated that over 50% of women over 40 years of age have the condition in varying degrees. In about 10% of patients who take the danazol androgen, a side effect is virilization or lowering of the voice.[15] The same drug is used in cases of severe endometriosis. Since there is as yet no clear indication whether voice changes are reversible, consultation between your gynecologist and a laryngologist is strongly advised in both instances.

Short-term Tissue Changes

The URI (Common Cold)

The most frequent cause of temporary tissue change is the ubiquitous upper respiratory infection (URI) or common cold. There is nothing at all common about it for the person who has one. Contrary to traditional wisdom, colds are transmitted by touch rather than by sneezing, coughing, or kissing so the best preventive measure is to wash the hands frequently and try to keep them away from the mouth and nose. If you do get a cold, proper treatment of the symptoms will make your week of misery a little easier.

Although the common cold is a viral infection, it opens the door to a series of bacterial infections, such as sinusitis, bronchitis, and laryngitis, all of which will probably incapacitate you for much longer than a week. The best treatment is to rest, increase fluid intake to at least ten glasses per day, and allow your own immune system to work its miracles. A room humidity between forty and fifty percent will keep mucus thin. During normal conditions, the body processes about a quart and a half of mucus each day, so if it becomes too thick and too little is produced, it irritates the pharynx and the vocal folds. The infamous post-nasal drip onto the cords is caused by mucus that is too thick and cannot be easily swallowed.

For some people, gargling with a saline solution of one-quarter teaspoon of salt and one-quarter teaspoon of soda in a cup of warm water relieves minor irritation in the pharynx. Although anesthetic sprays and lozenges are sometimes taken for a sore throat, they tend to numb nerve endings. Any medication which contains an ingredient with a "caine" suffix is an anesthetic. If an anesthetic spray or lozenge is used before a performance, the singer loses a sense of how much effort he/she is using.[16] All such preparations block the function of nerve endings and therefore cordal action cannot be safely monitored. Pain and/or an increase in body temperature is a symptom that something is wrong, and any substance which masks pain is an invitation to sing anyway and ignore the physical condition. In cases of severe bacterial infection, such as sinusitis, bring out the big guns and take the complete set of antibiotics prescribed by your doctor. For more severe throat conditions, a specialist should be consulted.

For those who believe in the magical powers of a whisky toddy, Dr. Brodnitz has words of warning.[17]

> People are seldom at loss for an excuse to take a drink, but in the case of an approaching cold, the belief in the germ-killing abilities of alcohol gives a special medical dignity to the consumption of a few drinks.

He goes on to say that alcohol actually dilates the blood vessels and upsets the heat balance of the body.

Vitamin C or antihistamines may be used during the first "wet" days, but both have a drying effect and more water intake is needed. Antihistamines in particular cause a thickening of mucus. Other preparations which have drying effects and block the normal action of salivary and mucous glands are nasal sprays and throat lozenges. In addition to the numbing effect mentioned above, sprays and lozenges, which provide only temporary relief, are habit forming because they circumvent normal body function. They also have a dehydrating effect because of their high acid content and their high sugar content, both of which thicken mucus.

The use of decongestants is a favored way of clearing congestion and inability to breathe freely. Even short-term use of these agents, however, causes a temporary fluid imbalance in the mucous membranes and resultant swelling of tissue. Gene Martin, a pharmacologist from the University of Kansas, says that " ... the excessive use of decongestants can cause a rebound congestion to occur and one can get into a vicious spiral with a pattern of continued and more frequent use of the agents in an attempt to control the side effect that is being caused by the agent itself."[18]

Similar conditions exist as a result of allergies, mold from ventilation ducts, and dust in rehearsal rooms and on stage. Many singers also experience nasal stuffiness and cold symptoms when in air conditioned surroundings. In addition to observing the do's and don't's described above, the advice of a good allergist will help pinpoint the problem.

Many singers feel a great need to "do something" about a cold. The best thing to do, of course, is to stay in bed for a day. Such a simple remedy, but not only will it shorten the life of your cold, it will prevent you from infecting others during the most contagious stage of this most common of illnesses.

Just a word about coughing. A continual, violent, hacking cough, generally experienced at the end of a URI, abuses the vocal folds. Especially at night, a cough suppressant may be the lesser of two evils. A milder cough is part of the body's self-cleaning action. "The vocal folds can stand a lot of mild coughing without harm."[19]

Tonsillitis

Tonsillitis or acute sore throat occurs when the tonsils and lymph glands of the neck become swollen and inflamed, making swallowing and/or talking painful. This condition generally is caused by bacteria and can be treated with antibiotics. The vocal cords may be red and swollen and the person nearly voiceless, or the upper surface of the cords may appear to be unaffected, while the lower surface and the trachea are bright red. The latter ailment is called tracheitis. One can sing for only a short time before the voice loses quality and decreases in intensity. Tracheitis generally lasts ten to fourteen days and is effectively treated with antibiotics.

If the tonsils are no longer functioning properly as protectors of the throat, but on the contrary, are chronically infected, surgery may be necessary. If, after at least two opinions by knowledgeable medical experts, a tonsillectomy is indicated, be sure that the surgeon is a specialist, not a jack-of-all-trades. For professional voice users, intubation with a plastic rather than a rubber tube is advised; it causes much less irritation.[20] After surgery, it generally takes from three to six months for the singing voice to return to normal.[21] The singer must expect a change in the shape of the vocal tract. How soon he/she will be comfortable with this "new" space seems to depend upon the individual and his/her kinesthetic awareness of pharyngeal dimensions.

Laryngitis

An especially severe, although temporary, tissue change takes place during acute laryngitis. The cause of the condition is generally an URI and can be either viral or bacterial. The mucous membranes of the vocal folds are extremely red and swollen, and this swelling causes increased heat and friction. Sometimes very little actual soreness is felt in the throat, but the person either cannot phonate at all or else the sound is husky, weak, and has frequent "breaks." Under these conditions, the vocal folds are extremely vulnerable to hemorrhages. Aspirin should not be taken because it thins the blood and might encourage hemorrhaging. It is best to observe as much silence as possible during a bout of laryngitis. Whispering is not advised. There is minimal cordal closure in the true whisper, but all too often the forced whisper is used instead. Since it is produced with extreme vocal fold tension and requires a lot of medial compression, it is a potentially damaging kind of phonation.

No singing should be done when any trace of laryngitis is present because this kind of vocal misuse can have long-lasting consequences. Frequently the singing voice appears normal, at least on first hearing, but the speaking voice evidences residual fuzziness. It is better to be conservative and postpone a full vocal workout until the vocal folds are completely healed. Sometimes a short lesson/warmup is reassuring so long as the goal is to reassure the singer that the voice is still there. Because singers are extremely verbal people, a strong warning about vocal rest is warranted.

The Effects of Drugs

Cortico-steroids are still a subject of much controversy. If a singer feels he/she must fulfill an important engagement and is suffering from swelling of the vocal folds such as was described above, should cortico-steroids be used to reduce the edema? In a panel discussion at the Twelfth Symposium on Care of the Professional Voice (1983), five doctors indicated what kind of cortico-steroid, in what form, when, and what dosage they would administer prior to a two-hour performance. Preferences were varied on all counts, and one of the five said he preferred not to use steroids at all, but might do so for "some exquisite emergency."[22] No matter how urgent that emergency may be, reduction of swelling by steroids is a risky business. Even if the cords are able to adduct, at least for the duration of the performance, the resultant sound is often thin and reedy and does not feel at all normal. There is distorted acoustical and kinesthetic feedback so that singers may be using too much cordal tension and/or too much subglottic pressure without knowing it. They are singing on a steroid and a prayer! Their professional reputations may suffer a severe blow, but even terrible reviews from major critics are not nearly so serious as the risk of permanent physical damage. Sataloff feels that if the laryngitis is severe enough to warrant a topical anesthetic, it is far better to cancel the performance.[23]

Of all non-prescription drugs, probably the most commonly used and one of the most dangerous is the amphetamine stimulant found in diet pills which suppress the appetite. This amphetamine is called phenylpropanolamine and is contained in **all** diet aids, no matter what the advertisements say.[24] It is a central nervous system stimulant.

Alcohol, barbituates, sedatives, and muscle relaxants such as diazepam (trade name: Valium) all have a negative influence on muscular coordination, particularly when used in large amounts. Any drug, whether a stimulant or a depressant, which prevents conscious control of fine muscle tone surely will influence the precise muscular timing necessary for singing.

In recent years there has been considerable interest in beta blockers to reduce the tremors of performance anxiety or stage fright. The most widely used is propranolol (trade name: Inderal). Epinephine, the chemical which is released by the adrenal glands during times of stress sometimes produces symptoms of "flight or fight," the most common of which are rapid heart beat, sweaty palm, dry mouth, tremors, the urge to urinate, and even nausea. Not all of these signs are felt by all or even a majority of performers. Propranolol is remarkably effective in blocking epinephine, and therefore reducing the heart rate, blood pressure, and nausea. Its effect upon mental alertness has not been documented, but it definitely reduces the adrenaline level. The use of beta blockers is advised by some authorities and condemned by others. It is certain, however, that they are potent drugs and should be taken only after consultation with a physician. It already has been established that they should not be taken by persons with such breathing disorders as asthma or with certain heart conditions.[25]

In addition to basic medical considerations, there is a broader issue. If pre-performance excitement and the accompanying adrenaline surge and increased heart beat are muted, is the ensuing passivity a desirable condition for performing? Perhaps it depends upon the severity of the stage fright symptoms. Still, the psychological and physical demands of the creative process are such that many of these unpleasant symptoms are probably indispensable prerequisites for a fully committed performance. Norman Punt says that one of the more comforting traditions of English actors and singers is the belief that Russian stout is an excellent drink while waiting for "curtain up."[26] Who knows, maybe stout is a safer and more enjoyable form of beta blocking.

Functional Disorders

Prolonged Phonation or Overuse

When does overuse become abuse? Like other athletes, vocal athletes are prone to injury. Because they are high achieving, strongly motivated performers, singers have a tendency to overwork the musculature, especially the adductors of the vocal folds. Titze says that the adductor-abductor muscles are among the fastest in the body so the risk of overusing them and causing tissue damage is always high.[27] One author calls this kind of overuse attempting to "exceed their natural functional capacity."[28]

By far the most common vocal misuse is overuse. Many singers do not even acknowledge that there **are** limits to the amount of time they should sing in a given day. It is a strange attitude because they will readily admit that there is a limit to how long they can run, swim, play tennis, or any number of other physical activities. Singing is no less taxing muscularly. Muscle tone declines and the ability of muscles to respond quickly and precisely is lost. Like any discrete set of muscles, the vocal folds in particular become sluggish. If daily overuse continues for a long period of time, permanent damage may be sustained.

Prolonged phonation at high frequencies is especially dangerous. When the breathing muscles are tired, the air stream becomes thin and under too much subglottic pressure, or else there is a fluctuating emission of air instead of a smooth, steady flow. In either case, breath, which acts as a cushion to protect and cool the cords, is inadequate. Thus efficient breath energy is impossible, and such inappropriate muscles as the false elevators and the root of the tongue take on the task. If the resulting tension becomes habitual, functional freedom is no longer possible.

In addition to fatigue of the vocal folds and the respiratory muscles, prolonged phonation increases the tissue viscosity of the former. Friction and dehydration increase.

Singers generally are gregarious people, and they like to talk. Since voice use is not confined to singing, singers need to be aware that their singing and speaking voices are not separate entities. Don't scream and yell at parties, football games, and similar events. Don't continually talk over noise. If you must speak, try to use a different frequency from the ambient noise and be sure to sound the consonants crisply for more intelligibility. Serious singers avoid situations in which continual loud talking is required, especially if they are tired or taking medication. This kind of excessive use when the cords are already irritated or when they are dry from certain drugs or from an allergic reaction is taking an unnecessary and foolish risk.

> The practice of singing three or four hours a day will ruin the most robust organ; three half hours a day at long intervals ought to be the maximum of study, and should give flexibility without risk of fatigue.[29]

Garcia's recommendation still holds true. The physical nature of the voice has not changed since his time. Even granting that vocal stamina increases with physical maturity, long-lived voices exceed one and one-half hours of singing per day only rarely. Few song recitals are longer, and opera roles generally require much less total singing time. Zinka Milanov sums up the issue of overuse.[30]

> Never give more than you have!
> That's the biggest illness for the voice.

"Marking"

For singers who understand that prolonged phonation is dangerous, the greatest frustration is long rehearsals for operas, musicals, or choral performances. Singers who are established professionals usually have control over the amount of time they rehearse, while students and pre-professionals do not. If they are lucky, the director of the opera or musical understands the singing voice and does not ask for full-voice production at every rehearsal. Because the singers are not fully trained in stage work, however, longer and more frequent rehearsals are often needed. Naturally, these young singers are most at risk because their instruments are not yet fully mature, nor is their technical training completed. They should be encouraged to "mark," a technique by which one sings softly in a normal voice without decreasing breath energy or air flow. Since soft singing often is difficult for young voices, marking must be taught.

It should not be assumed that if a young singer is asked to mark, he/she will know how to do it. Moderation and varying the modes of muscular action do not require nearly as much stamina as using those same muscles without any change in function. Listed below are a few basic guidelines for marking.

(1) Vary the dynamics and the "hook-up." Do not stint on air flow.
(2) Use frequent periods of talk-sing at approximate pitches. Stay in "character."
(3) Either avoid notes at both extremes of your range or sing them an octave lower or higher.
(4) Do not whistle or sing pianissimo for extended periods of time.
(5) Hum occasionally, but only for short periods. It is a relaxing device.
(6) If your neck muscles become tight or your throat is very tired, you may be sub-vocalizing. Even though you are not making a sound but merely

mouthing the words, your cords may be rubbing together.

(7) Practice various ways of marking during your studio lessons.

(8) Indicate various marking decisions in your score.

(9) Always tell the conductor and the other singers when you plan to mark.

Choral Singing

Choral singing presents its own problems. There is not much that a chorister can do about excessively long rehearsals other than to quit singing entirely. Often long rehearsals take place the day immediately preceding a concert. It is rather like cramming for an examination, since the percentage of musical or technical improvement is minuscule at such a late date, but the potential for vocal damage is great. Besides, if voices are overtaxed at rehearsals, the sound at the performance may be dull and lacking in vitality. If the piece being rehearsed is one with a lot of high, loud singing, such as in the Beethoven Ninth Symphony, the risk becomes intolerable, at least for choral conductors who understand their ethical responsibility toward the voices under their care.

Another factor in choral singing is that the majority of the singers cannot hear themselves, and consequently, they sing louder. The relationship between hearing the sound of one's own voice (feedback) and the sound of the rest of the choir (reference) is one of the most important acoustic factors in choral singing. There seems to be less masking by reference sound when placement of singers is mixed so that section colleagues are not standing next to each other. Various famous choral musicians have experimented with this concept. Unfortunately, intensity control is seldom monitored, particularly in large groups. There is double indemnity, therefore, if this kind of singing is combined with long rehearsals.

A 1988 study found that fundamental frequency precision deteriorated abruptly when reference sound is too loud.[31] The implications for good intonation are obvious. In a later study,[32] Ternström asked six experienced choir singers to sing sustained tones using a change of vowel in midtone. He then assembled data on which vowels affected the intonation of the sung tone and in what combinations. For more details of the study, the reader is referred to the article in the *Journal of Voice*. Suffice it to say that intonation was affected 63% of the time. If, however, appropriate vowel formants are reinforced, "sound pressure level (loudness) can be varied over a 25 decibel range without causing serious problems for fundamental frequency agreement in a choir."[33]

Choral singing should be an exciting and rewarding experience for young singers. If voices are treated with care and understanding, musical insight, technical growth, and creative fulfillment are possible. If the technical aspect is neglected, however, the basic prerequisite for a lifetime of singing is missing.

All choral rehearsals should begin with at least ten minutes of vocalization. Warming up voices by singing a piece currently under study not only neglects the technical development of the choristers, but also places no emphasis upon the need to listen to each other. For groups of fifty or less, a regular voice training session in vocal techniques is time well spent. In a very short time, the results will be heard in the overall balance and blend of the group.

A word of caution. If you are conducting a choir, do not sing with the group and especially do not sing all four parts in rehearsals. Such behavior is almost as vocally abusive as becoming a cheerleader. Besides, your singers will become more independent and will not face the temptation of imitating your vocal color if your musical indications are non-verbal.

Some voice scientists support those singing teachers who believe that certain solo singers should not sing in choral groups.[34] Those very characteristics which make some solo voices unique must be subdued in group singing, often to the eventual detriment of that voice. In solo singing, sopranos generally produce more energy in the 2000-4000 cps range, although there are individual differences in the sound spectra in this range.[35] If a voice has a unique color and/or a high degree of ring, whether because of the singing formant or because of the acoustical advantage of high frequencies, it will not blend easily unless vocal fold adduction is reduced. Generally the extent of the vibrato also must be reduced from that used in solo singing. That singer then may be singing at half-voice, not a condition conducive to functional freedom if continued for any length of time. If the color is altered as well, the voice may never regain its former "bloom."

Knowledgeable choral conductors encourage singing that relies on the ring of the singing formant to project the sound, rather than emphasizing only the fundamental and the lower partials. The latter sound is easier to blend with other voices, but the overall sound is flat and non-resonant.

> There is no reason to have a Stradivarius sound like a cigar-box violin so that both will sound the same. ... The great orchestras are built on the great techniques of the individuals in the organization--certainly the greatest choirs will operate with this philosophy since the coloring would be more varied and communicative.[36]

In light of the extremely complex nature of the singing voice, we must always remember that no one has all the answers. Given a basic knowledge of the physical and acoustical parameters of this instrument, it is wise to practice tolerance of other methods of teaching singing until the end product, the sound, is heard. Do not make judgments based solely upon faculty hearsay or student anecdotes. If the private voice teacher and the choral musician are true professionals and hold each other in high regard, differing viewpoints can be explored and an avenue of communication established. The young singers in our charge will be the beneficiaries of this respectful, understanding atmosphere.

The Wrong Tessitura

Unfortunately, singing voices are sometimes classified as early as junior high school, particularly female voices. At that age there rarely is any difference in quality between the soprano and alto voices, but all too often the stronger singers or those girls who can sight read the harmony part are categorized as altos. The pattern is set, and from then on they are "trained" as altos. Young singers should not be permitted to sing at inappropriate tessituras merely because more voices are needed in that section. Because of the nature of mutation in adolescent males, however, they are less likely to be put in a specific classification and kept there. Still, a young bass may eventually become a baritone or even a tenor, and a consistent program of voice testing is essential because the tessitura changes so rapidly. In high school, few males sing to F^4 with ease; an upper limit of C^4 or D^4 is more common, especially for the bigger voices.

Contrary to popular opinion, young female voices are most at risk because changes in tessitura are harder to detect. It is extremely important to keep these young voices flexible by eliminating excessive weight and maintaining a good balance of head and chest registers. Bright timbre works best when the muscles are still immature. An unnaturally dark timbre often creates tension in the root of the tongue and excessive subglottic pressure. The belting style so prevalent in musicals creates even more tension and there is no control of intensity levels. The vocalis is overworked, there is no balance of resonances, breath pressure is too high and the tone is straight. These conditions indicate a state of severe vocal misuse. Added to all these danger signs is the unduly low tessitura. Although the tessitura in a few musicals is at a moderate level, in many more of them it rests between F^3 and C^4. Voice therapists do a thriving business because of the harmful demands made upon untrained, developing adolescent voices.

The Young Voice

This seems an appropriate place to talk about what we mean by the young voice. Yes, we mean junior high school and high school voices. In these voices, barely past puberty, the macro muscles work, but the micro muscles are in a very early developmental stage. Vocal stability is particularly difficult for male singers because vocal mutation for the singing voice, although usually completed in six months, can take as long as three years.[37] Since there is great irregularity in muscle development in both males and females, there is generally a lot of difference between individuals and even within an individual from day to day. The tone is often breathy (mutational chink) in both sexes, although this symptom is more common in females.

What is sometimes not well understood is that college age voices are also in the process of anatomical maturation. Laryngeal development is not complete until the late 20s or early 30s.[38]

The single most important trait of the young voice is its limited endurance. For the high school voice, the medium dynamic level is best. Very soft or very loud singing, except for a limited time is not advised. The tessitura must be carefully monitored, even for college age singers, and singing for too long a time is especially dangerous. Always exercise overcaution rather than undercaution.

The Aging Voice

> One of the most robust findings in aging research is the extreme individual variation with which motor performance decline occurs.[39]

Just as there are 60-year-old marathon runners, there are singers like the legendary Giuseppe de Luca who sang until he was 70 and the legendary Alfredo Kraus (b. 1927) who is still singing with seemingly undiminished resources. In contrast, the child-belter or the rock singer or the operatic singer with an inadequate, abusive technique may show a warn-out, geriatric voice at 30 years of age. Indeed, it is Sataloff's opinion that it is much more difficult to rehabilitate a child singer who has sung abusively for a long period of time than an adult with similar habits who is motivated to change.[40] The physiological difference between the two is that the muscles of the child singer have been shaped when in their young, developmental stages and therefore have a tendency to maintain that shape for a long time. Once again, we see what an ethical responsibility singing teachers have to insure that young singers get a dependable technical start.

In addition to a reliable, healthy technique, an equally important factor is one's physiological condition. It is probable that such considerations as weight, blood pressure, percentage of body fat, and breathing vital capacity are even more important than chronological age, and that vocal deterioration, like other kinds of physical decline, can be held back by a healthful life style, nutrition, and exercise. For the singer, exercise definitely means regular vocalization. As we all know, we can get away with less and less in terms of technique as we get older.[41] Keeping in good shape with cardiovascular exercise is especially crucial for the older singer. Muscular strength is relatively easy to maintain in comparison with cardiovascular efficiency.

Hirano et al.[42] found that in older men, the layers of the lamina propria of the vocal folds show greater changes in thickness and elasticity than in older women. There is no mention of the health habits or professions of the owners of these excised larynxes. It is interesting to note, however, that many of the studies on the aging voice are especially concerned about the effects of menopause on the female voice, although it is probably impossible to separate normal wear-

and-tear non-hormonal factors from possible changes in hormonal balance.

An intriguing 1987 study (Morris and Brown) employed 25 women 20-35 years of age and 25 women over 75 years of age. All were normal, healthy women; none had vocal pathologies. Results showed no significant difference in vocal effort (intensity and subglottic pressure) between the two groups.[43] The only consistent difference was in longer phoneme duration of both vowels and consonants for the older group. Is this less precise articulaton the result of social expectations? Or is it an age-related slowing of transmissions by the nervous system? Perhaps more research on the normal aging voice will provide answers, but the variability of subjects will present difficulties. Just as mutational changes in the adolescent voice sometimes do not proceed according to expectation, so changes in the aging voice do not occur at a uniform rate. Thus far we have been unable to define "aging voice" by chronological age. Like Nolan Ryan, still pitching successfully in the major leagues at 45 years of age, take the high road, get on with it, and just do it!

Am I Too Loud?

Are you trying to sing over
amplified instruments?

Were you tired before you started singing,
but are giving all you've got anyway?

Do you always try as hard as
you can when you're singing?

If the answer to any of these questions is yes, you are using too much force. Often we have specific images of range and tone color based on what we want to sound like. Rarely do these images coincide with reality, but since intellectual conceptions are very strong, we think we hear the sounds we want to produce. Hyperfunction, too much muscular force, is particularly harmful because hypertension and hyperfunction go hand in hand.

A classic example of hyperfunction is the cheerleader. Her concept of "conversational level" is much higher than the norm among adult females. During actual cheerleading, the sound pressure level is close to maximal, indicating the probable presence of excessive laryngeal muscular effort, inefficient vocal fold adduction and a very constricted lower airway system operating on small resonance cavities.[44] The functional imbalance is similar to that found during forceful belting, which is an abusive and inefficient practice; vocal fold irritation is inevitable. A long-term prognosis depends upon individual physical characteristics and how deep-seated this behavior has become.

Rubin issues a strong warning to singers when he says that excessive volume combined with a basically good vocal technique can be as destructive to the laryngeal muscles as poor technique alone.[45]

Weird Noises

Using an unnatural vocal quality leads to vocal dysfunction; it is abusive behavior. Screaming and yelling at a sports event results in obvious and almost immediate symptoms that are similar to acute laryngitis. If this kind of phonation is occupational, as in the case of the cheerleader or the auctioneer, prolonged strain causes permanent damage.

More gradual symptoms may occur if you do your Donald Duck imitation at every party you attend. Comedy singers and actors also must use care in how certain sounds are produced and at what tessitura. Those who have long careers and suffer little or no vocal dysfunction understand what kinds of vocal production are potentially dangerous and how to use air flow and nasal resonance to avoid undue strain.

Untrained comics, comedy singers, and imitators are not even aware of the dangers, let alone the precautions that are needed. In addition to using ample air flow and nasal resonance, do not sing or talk too long on one breath. Forced breathing and muscular hyperfunction feed upon each other and tension in the vocal cords, throat, and tongue increase.

Extended Vocal Techniques

Of special interest to singers are some of the unusual sounds called for in avant garde music. Vowels can and should be altered and tonal weight lightened when singing extremely wide intervals. Titze estimates that "a 2-octave (4:1) change in fundamental frequency requires a 16:1 change in muscle stress."[46] How much better, then to increase air flow and sing with more light mechanism in the sound.

Another important aspect of this kind of singing is how to handle clicks, pops, barks, snaps, and similar plosive sounds. Let us say that the duration of the piece is ten minutes, and, in addition to the lyrics, the singer is asked to imitate the sounds of a pinball machine or a helicopter. If the cords are allowed to vibrate at will while these sounds are produced under very high breath pressure, the singer will feel the effects for a long time afterward and may be unable to phonate clearly for days or even weeks. If, however, the cords are closed, using only the movement of the articulators and the air in the vocal tract, projection will be adequate and irritation of the vocal folds minimized.

As a final admonition, avoid as much as possible those pieces for female singers in which the text is set syllabically. Unless the composer understands vowel formants, he/she is likely to set the text at a high tessitura, regardless of how many closed front vowels are used. If there are melismas, however, intelligibility and ease of production will increase substantially.

NOTES

1. F. S. Brodnitz, *Vocal Rehabilitation* (Rochester, Minn.: Whiting Press, 1967), 47.

2. Robert Thayer Sataloff, "The Professional Voice: Part III. Common Diagnoses & Treatments," *Journal of Voice*, 1:3 (1987), 284.

3. M. Hirano lecture at Biology of Music Making Conference, Denver Center for the Performing Arts, July 10, 1984. See also M. Hirano, S. Kurita, K. Matsuo, and K. Nagata, "Laryngeal Tissue Reaction to Stress," *Care of the Professional Voice*, Transcripts of the Ninth Symposium, Part II (New York: Voice Foundation, 1980), 15.

4. M. Hirano, "Vocal Mechanisms in Singing: Laryngeal and Phoniatric Aspects," *Journal of Voice*, 2:1 (1988), 51-69.

5. Minoru Hirano, "Morphological Structure of the Vocal Cord as a Vibrator and Its Variations," *Folia Phoniatrica*, 26:2 (1974), 89-94.

6. Hirano, et al., "Laryngeal Tissue," op. cit., 15.

7. Robert J. Feder, M.D., lecture at the Fourteenth Symposium on Care of the Professional Voice, Denver, Colorado, June 12, 1985.

8. Daniel R. Boone, *The Voice and Voice Therapy* (Englewood Cliffs, N.J.: Prentice-Hall, 1971), 55-56.

9. Björn Fritzell, "Singing and the Health of the Voice," *Research Aspects on Singing* (Stockholm: Royal Swedish Academy of Music, 1981), 99. See also Norman A. Punt, *The Singer's and Actor's*

Throat (London: William Heinemann, 1951), 53.

10. Punt, op. cit., 54.

11. Hirano, et al., "Laryngeal Tissue," op. cit., 12.

12. Thomas Watterson, Heidi J. Hansen-Magorian, and Stephen C. McFarlane, "A Demographic Description of Laryngeal Contact Ulcer Patients," *Journal of Voice*, 4:1 (1990), 75.

13. Nicolas E. Maragos, "Complications of Endotracheal Intubation in the Singer," *Care of the Professional Voice*, Transcripts of the Tenth Symposium, Part II (New York: Voice Foundation, 1981), 151.

14. Jean Abitbol, Jean de Brux, Ginette Millot, Marie-Francoise Masson, Odile Languille Mimoun, Helene Pau, and Beatrice Abitbol, "Does a Hormonal Cord Cycle Exist in Women? Study of Vocal Premenstral Syndrome in Voice Performers by Videostroboscopy-Glottography and Cytology on 38 Women," *Journal of Voice*, 3:2 (1989), 157-162.

15. Colton and Casper, op. cit., 89.

16. E. Gene Martin, "Drugs and the Voice," *Care of the Professional Voice*, Transcripts of the Twelfth Symposium, Part I (New York: Voice Foundation, 1983), 135.

17. Brodnitz, *Keep Your Voice*, op. cit., 83.

18. Martin, op. cit., 127.

19. Brodnitz, *Keep Your Voice*, op. cit., 115.

20. Robert Thayer Sataloff, "The Professional Voice: Part I. Anatomy, Function, and General Health," *Journal of Voice*, 1:1 (1987), 101.

21. Ibid., 101-102.

22. Panel Discussion, *Care of the Professional Voice*, Transcripts of the Twelfth Symposium, Part I, Van Lawrence, ed. (New York: Voice Foundation, 1983), 141-142.

23. Robert Thayer Sataloff, "The Professional Voice: Part III. Common Diagnoses and Treatments," *Journal of Voice*, 1:3 (1987), 288.

24. Martin, op. cit., 125.

25. Ibid., 131.

26. Punt, op. cit., 84.

27. Ingo Titze, "Pressed Voice: A Problem for Singers and Speakers," *NATS Journal*, 43:3 (1987), 22.

28. M. Stuart Strong, "Work-Related Injuries of Professional Singers: Their Significance and Management," Chapter 42, *Vocal Physiology: Voice Production, Mechanisms, and Functions*, Opamu Fujimura, ed. (New York: Raven Press, 1988), 462.

29. Garcia, *Hints*, op. cit., 18.

30. Jerome Hines, *Great Singers on Great Singing*, (Garden City, NY: Doubleday, 1982), 171.

31. Sten Ternström and Johan Sundberg, "Intonation Precision of Choir Singers," *Journal of the Acoustical Society of America*, 84:1 (1988), 59-69.

32. Sten Ternström, "Physical and Acoustic Factors that Interact with the Singer to Produce the Choral Sound," *Journal of Voice*, 5:2 (1991), 128-143.

33. Ternström and Sundberg, "Intonation Precision," op. cit., 69.

34. Thomas D. Rossing, Johan Sundberg, and Sten Ternström, "Acoustic Comparison of Voice Use in Solo and Choir Singing," *Journal of Acoustical Society of America*, 79:6 (1986), 1981.

35. Thomas D. Rossing, Johan Sundberg, and Sten Ternström, "Acoustic Comparison of Soprano Solo and Choir Singing," *Journal of the Acoustical Society of America*, 82:3 (1987), 836.

36. Coffin, *Sounds of Singing*, op. cit., p. 166.

37. Robert T. Sataloff and Joseph R. Spiegel, "The Young Voice," *NATS Journal*, 45:3 (1989), 36.

38. Leon Thurman and Van Lawrence, "Voice Care for Vocal Athletes in Training," *Choral Journal*, 20:9 (1980), 34-35, 56.

39. Robert L. Ringel and Wojtek J. Chodzko-Zajko, "Vocal Indices of Biological Age," *Journal of Voice*, 1:1 (1987), 31.

40. John F. Michel, Robert Coleman, Leslie Guinn, Diane Bless, Craig Timberlake, and Robert T. Sataloff, "Aging Voice: Panel 2," *Journal of Voice*, 1:1 (1987), 66.

41. Ibid., Sataloff, 62.

42. Minoru Hirano, Shigejiro Kurita, and Shinji Sakaguchi, "Aging of the Vibratory Tissue of Human Vocal Folds," *Acta Otolaryngolica*, 107:5/6 (1989), 428-433.

43. Richard J. Morris and W. S. Brown, Jr., "Age-Related Voice Measures Among Adult Women," *Journal of Voice*, 1:1 (1987), 42.

44. M. A. McHenry and A. R. Reich, "Effective Airway Resistance and Vocal Sound Pressure Level in Cheerleaders with a History of Dysphonic Episodes," *Folia Phoniatrica*, 37:5 (1985), 230-231.

45. Henry J. Rubin, "Role of the Laryngologist in Management of Dysfunctions of the Singing Voice," *NATS Bulletin*, 22:4 (1966), 22.

46. Ingo R. Titze, "Fundamental Frequency Scaling and Voice Classification," *NATS Bulletin*, 37:1 (1980), 21.

Appendix II

VOCAL HYGIENE

Common Irritants

A 1990 study of 352 subjects found that house dust produced an allergic reaction more frequently than any other common agent, although house dust generally is not thought of as a specific allergen per se.[1] Imagine then how at risk the singer is. Backstage facilities are rarely cleaned and curtains, whether in dressing rooms or on stage, often are repositories for years of dust. Short of adding "charwoman" or "janitor" to the job description on your contract, there is not much to be done. Since many buildings, whether concert halls, theaters, churches, or homes, use forced air heating or some other very drying system, a humidifier is almost a necessity. It also helps to settle the dust. Another "must" is relative voice rest outside the theater and knowing how to mark. Both are as effective as any drug you might take.

Other common irritants in today's urban society are air pollutants and passive smoke. It is probable that one is subject to a higher percentage of infections as a result. There is no solution to the air pollution situation except to support stronger regulation of automobile, truck, and industrial emissions. Passive smoke is much more of a problem for those who sing in night clubs than for opera and concert singers. In recent years it has become easier to find a restaurant that bans smoking entirely.

Smoke of any kind is extremely irritating and dries out the tissues of the nose and throat. Heat from a cigarette has been measured at 300°-400° F. in the mouth, considerably above the boiling point of water.[2] Marijuana smoke is even hotter because the paper burns at such high heat. Cocaine, in addition to its addictive properties, irritates the nasal tissues, dries up mucus, and alters sensory perception.

If a food allergy is suspected, see an allergist for tests. If every time you eat a chocolate bar, your nose becomes stuffed up, there is no need for a doctor's diagnosis. The same is true for those singers who are allergic to dog or cat hair. No chocolate and no pets may reduce the quality of your life, but at least you know what your choices are.

The kinds of irritation discussed above can signal a change in the throat that takes only three to five minutes to accomplish. Possible vocal effects are (1) breathiness because the glottis remains partially open, (2) decreased intensity, and (3) a husky, muffled quality.

Commonly Used Drugs

Although we spoke in Appendix I of drugs used for short term tissue changes such as laryngitis and the URI, there was not enough emphasis there on the harmful side effects of certain drugs.

Granted, cortico-steroids do reduce muscle bulk or swelling of the vocal folds, but they also suppress the immune system and encourage water retention.[3]

Long term use of decongestants results in a "decongestant habit" and may even create lesions in the nasal mucous membrane because of consistent reduction of blood flow to the tissues.[4] Short-term use of cough suppressants, expectorants, antihistamines, and antispasmotics for gastrointestinal problems should be accompanied by drinking a lot of water. If you can, find a cough suppressant without antihistamine. Martin finds that wetting agents or expectorants often contain cough suppressants as well and advises the use of those containing only giuafenesin.[5] The most common such over-the-counter preparation is Robitussin.

Hydration

Lack of sufficient saliva and mucus, the dry mouth and throat syndrome, is especially noticeable during performances, but certainly is not confined to those occasions. If the nose and the salivary glands manufacture about a quart and a half of saliva and thin mucus every day, this fluid must be replaced. Further loss of fluid occurs from the waste products of the body. Water, then is of great importance for proper functioning of the respiratory system and the vocal tract. When the vocal folds vibrate and rub against each other, friction and heat are generated. The wider the amplitude of vibration, the higher the intensity level and the greater the friction. No wonder the sustained phonation of loud high notes is the high road to vocal fatigue. This increased viscosity can be reduced by insuring that the vocal folds are well lubricated. Fluid intake can be directly deposited on the folds, but even more important is the internal irrigation system.

The phonation threshold level or the lung pressure needed to start the vibration of the vocal folds is lowest under wet vocal fold conditions, regardless of whether the person is a trained professional voice user or not. The other two factors affecting the lung pressure needed most directly are the viscosity or stickiness, often alleviated by increased hydration, and how high the fundamental frequency.[6]

Drink at least eight full glasses of water per day. Use a humidifier, particularly in your bedroom. Between forty and fifty percent humidity is preferred, and thirty percent is the minimum needed. Since steam ionizes water molecules which ultimately results in dehydration, use a cold water humidifier. The low humidity common in the winter may be one reason why colds are more prevalent then.

When traveling by air, be particularly careful to drink more water than usual. Do not drink alcohol, a drying agent in itself, or iced drinks. Even soft drinks, which contain sugar or other sweeteners, thicken mucus. Some travelers keep a moist towel over the nose and mouth during flight. Since the humidity in planes can be as low as 10%, any kind of humidity enhancement will help reduce the amount of vocal fold recovery time needed at the end of the flight.[7] Another danger during air travel is the cabin noise level. At such high ambient noise levels, conversational speech can become abusively loud. All but absolutely necessary talking should be avoided.

Rest and Exercise

Basic to a singer's life of vigorous physical activity are an appropriate non-competitive exercise program and plenty of rest. The one thing that an athlete cannot do without is rest, particularly the night before a game or a performance.

Getting enough rest in the jet age is a juggling act at best. Leonie Rysanek arrives in a city two weeks before she is scheduled to sing, while Alfredo Kraus warns against singing in two cities on successive days because "your subconscious is working in both places, and it's too busy."[8] In addition to one's subconscious, the singer must adjust to a new altitude and a new time zone. Both require more than a few hurried hours of acclimation. Brodnitz says that horses which are brought up from the plains to the mountains refuse to canter until they adapt to their new environment.[9]

Allied to the subject of air travel, of course, is the tendency to block out too ambitious a schedule. Whether a professional, a pre-professional, or a student, a regimen of multiple jobs, auditioning, studying acting and dance, coaching new roles, and attending long rehearsals almost presupposes not enough rest. Sometimes the professional singer must long for the time when there were few summer festivals and opera productions, and singers spent the summer resting and learning new roles. The advanced student or pre-professional is especially susceptible to too much activity without enough rest.

Another kind of rest, vocal rest, is mandatory **after** a performance. Naturally, the vocal folds are slightly swollen after such strenuous activity, and, like the baseball pitcher's arm, they need and deserve several days of rest.

Individual tastes differ about exercise. Some singers prefer regular swimming, a bilateral and relatively gentle activity. Others do stretching and range of motion drills with light weights, a good way to encourage flexibility and fluidity of motion. Heavy weight lifting is not recommended.

The most important word in the above paragraph is "regular." No matter how busy your schedule, the benefits of physical exercise, like vocalizing, depend upon a consistent program.

Clothing and Diet

Daily changes in weather require attention to proper clothing. Singers too often dress too warmly. The layered protection of shirts, sweaters, and jackets which can be put on or taken off as temperature, humidity, wind, and heated buildings justify is the most practical solution. Since physically the main function of clothing is to provide an insulating layer of air around the body, clothes that are too heavy generally invite more colds than they help avoid. Brodnitz thinks that men wear too much clothing and points to tight belts, shirts with tight collars, and too many layers of clothing.[10] The looser clothing of recent years is certainly an improvement, as is the decreased use of neckties or ones tied so loosely that they should more properly be called scarves. When possible, light, informal clothing is best.

Opinions vary widely on what "sensible" means in relation to what one eats. For the person who enjoys fresh fruits and vegetables, whole-grain breads, and fish, giving up sweets and starches is no problem. Since most singers love to eat, though, a big spaghetti dinner topped off with chocolate mousse is heaven. Certain matters should be mentioned here. First of all, fat singers are a thing of the past on the world's concert and opera stages. With few exceptions, public taste demands that singers look like the characters they portray. Secondly, eating too much and drinking late at night after a performance generally mean a poor night's sleep, unwelcome extra weight, and perhaps even a bout with gastroesophageal reflux. Finally, milk products, chocolate, and soft drinks coat the throat and add a layer of mucus so do not indulge in them before a performance.

Emotional Stress

The singing voice is an instrument which is activated as much by mental and emotional elements as by physical ones. Although this book has described at some length the functional interdependence of the physical instrument, mental and emotional factors are equally important parts of a singer's total persona.

The effects of anxiety and emotional stress on physical function can be devastating. Since a singer's concept of self cannot be separated from his/her instrument, it is no wonder that emotional stress is instantly transmitted into disturbances in the vocal organs. Temporary anxiety, such as stage fright, produces fear, nervousness, and inhibitions, all of which show up in reduced respiratory efficiency and increased muscular tension. To performing anxiety can be added the effects of adverse reviews and failed auditions. Almost all performers remember the cracked high note, the memory slip, or the one negative comment by the audition judge more than successfully singing a difficult role or winning a competition. To help alleviate the symptoms and the anxiety triggering them, neck and back massage, lots of tender loving care and assurances of worth, and supervised vocal warm-ups are suggested. The latter may convince the singer that "the voice" really is still there. Those singers who have a sense of security about their vocal techniques seldom succumb to severe stage fright, regardless of the provocation. For chronic anxiety and stress, psychiatric counseling is indicated, together with training in biofeedback techniques.

Can one really separate physical stress from psychological stress? Probably not. Let us first take to heart, then, the value of rest, hydration, exercise, and the other daily habits mentioned earlier. Handling other kinds of stress will be that much easier if we are in top physical shape.

All successful singing teachers also recognize the importance of semantics in dealing with emotional stress. Titze[11] calls comfort words such as freedom and enjoyment combined with energy words like vitality and buoyancy important aids for alleviating stress. Perhaps these encouraging words will bring about a truly expressive singing of a special song. At other times, just listening to a student will clear his or her mind, and the way is open for the healing power of the music itself.

NOTES

1. Marja-Leena Haapanen, "Provoked Laryngeal Dysfunction," *Folia Phoniatrica*, 42:4 (1990), 157-169.

2. Van L. Lawrence, "Cigarettes and Whiskey and Wild, Wild Women," *NATS Bulletin*, 38:3 (1982), 27.

3. T. M. Harris, "The Pharmacological Treatment of Voice Disorders," *Folia Phoniatrica*, 44:3/4 (1992), 146.

4. F. Gene Martin, "Drugs and Vocal Function," *Journal of Voice*, 2:4 (1988), 341.

5. Ibid., 342.

6. Katherine Verdolini-Marston, Ingo R. Titze, and David G. Druker, "Changes in Phonation Threshold Pressure with Induced Conditions of Hydration," *Journal of Voice*, 4:2 (1990), 142-151.

7. Robert J. Feder, "Singing and Flying," *NATS Bulletin*, 41:1 (1984), 26.

8. Quoted by Martha Duffy in "Why Golden Voices Fade," *Time*, May 6, 1991, 75.

9. Brodnitz, *Keep Voice*, op. cit., 70.

10. Ibid., 71.

11. Ingo Titze, "A Word about Words," *NATS Journal*, 45:4 (1989), 19.

BIBLIOGRAPHY

BOOKS

Alexander, F. Matthias. *Man's Supreme Inheritance.* New York: E.P. Dutton, 1918.

_________. *The Universal Constant in Living*, 1st ed. New York: E.P. Dutton, 1941.

Andrews, Moya L., and Anne C. Summers. *Voice Therapy for Adolescents.* San Diego: Singular Publ. Group, 1991 [Reprint of 1988 ed.].

Appelman, D. Ralph. *The Science of Vocal Pedagogy*, 1st Midland ed. Bloomington, Indiana: Indiana University Press, 1986.

Askill, John. *Physics of Musical Sounds.* New York: D. Van Nostrand Co., 1979.

Bachner, Louis. *Dynamic Singing.* London: D. Dobson, 1947.

Backus, John. *The Acoustical Foundations of Music*, 2nd ed. New York: W.W. Norton, 1977.

Baer, Thomas, Clarence Sasaki, and Katherine S. Harris, eds. *Laryngeal Function in Phonation and Respiration.* Boston: College-Hill Press, 1987.

Bartholomew, Wilmer T. *Acoustics of Music.* Westport, Conn.: Greenwood Press, 1980 [Reprint of 1952 ed.].

Basmajian, John V. *Primary Anatomy*, 8th ed. Baltimore: Williams & Wilkins, 1982.

Benade, Arthur H. *Fundamentals of Musical Acoustics.* New York: Dover Publ., 1990 [Reprint of 1976 ed.].

Bérard, Jean-Baptiste. *L'art du chant*, translated by Sidney Murray. Milwaukee: Pro Musica Press, 1969 [Reprint of 1775 ed.].

Bless, Diane M., and James H. Abbs, eds. *Vocal Fold Physiology: Contemporary Research and Clinical Issues*. San Diego: College-Hill Press, 1983.

Boone, Daniel R. *The Voice and Voice Therapy*. Englewood Cliffs, N.J.: Prentice-Hall, 1971.

Borden, Gloria J., and Katherine S. Harris. *Speech Science Primer*. Baltimore: Williams & Wilkins, 1980.

Bouhuys, Arend, ed. *Sound Production in Man*. New York: New York Academy of Sciences, 1968.

Brodnitz, Friedrich S. *Keep Your Voice Healthy*. Boston: College-Hill Press, 1991 [Reprint of 1988 ed.].

__________. *Vocal Rehabilitation*. Rochester, Minn.: Whiting, 1967.

Brown, W. E. *Vocal Wisdom: Maxims of G. B. Lamperti*. Reprint. New York: Arno Press, 1968.

Browne, Lennox, and Emil Behnke. *Voice, Song, and Speech*. London: Samson Low, Marston, Searle, and Rivington, 1887.

Bunch, Meribeth. *Dynamics of the Singing Voice*. New York: Springer-Verlag, 1982.

Burgin, John Carroll. *Teaching Singing*. Metuchen, N.J.: Scarecrow Press, 1973.

Caruso, Enrico, and Luisa Tetrazzini. *Caruso and Tetrazzini on the Art of Singing*. New York: Dover Publications, 1975 [Reprint of 1909 ed.].

Chiba, Tsutomu, and Masato Kajiyama. *The Vowel: Its Nature and Structure.* Tokyo: Phonetic Society of Japan, 1958.

Coffin, Berton. *Coffin's Overtones of Bel Canto*, 1st ed. Metuchen, N.J.: Scarecrow Press, 1980.

_________. *Historical Vocal Pedagogy Classics.* Metuchen, N.J.: Scarecrow Press, 1989.

_________. *The Sounds of Singing*, 2nd ed. Metuchen, N.J.: Scarecrow Press, 1987.

Colton, Raymond H., and Janina K. Casper. *Understanding Voice Problems: a Physiological Perspective for Diagnosis and Treatment.* Baltimore: Williams & Wilkins, 1990.

Cooper, Morton. *Change Your Voice, Change Your Life.* New York: Macmillan Publishing, 1984.

_________. *Modern Techniques of Vocal Rehabilitation.* Springfield, IL: C.C. Thomas, 1973.

Cooper, Morton, and Marcia Hartung Cooper, eds. *Approaches to Vocal Rehabilitation.* Springfield, IL: C.C. Thomas, 1977.

Culver, Charles A. *Musical Acoustics*, 4th ed. New York: McGraw-Hill, 1956.

Denes, Peter B., and Elliot N. Pinson. *The Speech Chain: The Physics and Biology of Spoken Language.* Garden City, N.Y.: Anchor Press, 1963.

Dickson, David Ross, and Wilma Maue-Dickson. *Anatomical and Physiological Bases of Speech*, 1st ed. Boston: Little, Brown, 1982.

Duey, Philip A. *Bel Canto in Its Golden Age: A Study of Its Teaching Concepts*. New York: Da Capo Press, 1980 [Reprint of 1951 ed.].

Fant, Gunnar. *Acoustic Theory of Speech Production*. The Hague: Mouton, 1960.

Fields, Victor Alexander. *Foundations of the Singer's Art*, 2nd ed. Jacksonville, FL: National Association of Teachers of Singing, 1984.

_________. *Training the Singing Voice*. New York: Da Capo Press, 1979 [Reprint of 1947 ed.].

Fillebrown, Thomas. *Resonance in Singing and Speaking*, 3rd ed. Boston: Oliver Ditson, ca. 1911.

Fletcher, Harvey. *Speech and Hearing in Communication* [2nd ed.] New York: D. Van Nostrand, 1953.

Foote, Jeffrey. *The Vocal Performer: Development through Science and Imagery*. Mt. Pleasant, MI: Wildwood Music, 1980.

Franca, Ida. *Manual of Bel Canto*. New York: Coward-McCann, 1959.

Frisell, Anthony. *The Baritone Voice*. Boston: Crescendo Publications, 1972.

_________. *The Soprano Voice*. Boston: B. Humphries, 1966.

_________. *The Tenor Voice*. Boston: B. Humphries, 1964.

Fry, D. B., ed. *Acoustic Phonetics*. London: Cambridge University Press, 1976.

Fuchs, Victor H. *The Art of Singing and Voice Technique*. New York: London House & Maxwell, 1964.

Fucito, Salvatore, and Barnet J. Beyer. *Caruso and the Art of Singing*. New York: F.A. Stokes, 1929.

Fujimura, Osamu, ed. *Vocal Fold Physiology: Voice Production, Mechanisms and Functions*. New York: Raven Press, 1988.

Garcia, Manuel. *The Art of Singing, Part I*. Boulder, CO: Milton Enterprises, 1968 [Reprint of the 1840 ed.].

_________. *A Complete Treatise on the Art of Singing, Part II* (editions of 1847 and 1872), translated and edited by Donald V. Paschke. New York: Da Capo Press, 1975.

_________. *Hints on Singing*, translated by Beata Garcia. London: Ascerberg, Hopwood, and Crew, 1894.

Gauffin, Jan, and Britta Hammarberg, eds. *Vocal Fold Physiology: Acoustic, Perceptual, and Physiological Aspects of Voice Mechanisms*. San Diego: Singular Publishing Group, 1991.

Gelb, Michael. *Body Learning: An Introduction to the Alexander Technique*. New York: H. Holt, 1987 [Reprint of the 1981 ed.].

Gray, Henry. *Gray's Anatomy*, Rev. American, from the 15th English ed., edited by T. Pickering Pick and Robert Howden. New York: Bounty Books, 1977.

Hall, Donald E. *Musical Acoustics: An Introduction*. Belmont, California: Wadsworth Publishing, 1980.

Hamilton, Clarence G. *Sound and Its Relation to Music*. Boston: Oliver Ditson, 1912.

Helmholtz, Hermann L. F. *On the Sensations of Tone, as a Physiological Basis for the Theory of Music*, 2nd English ed., translated from the 4th German ed. of 1877, by Alexander J. Ellis. New York: Dover Publications, 1954.

Henderson, W. J. *The Art of Singing*. Freeport, N.Y.: Books for Libraries Press, 1938.

Herbert-Caesari, Edgar F. *The Science and Sensations of Vocal Tone*. Boston: Crescendo Publ., 1971 [Reprint of 1936 ed.].

_________. *The Voice of the Mind*. London: Robert Hale, 1963.

Hines, Jerome. *Great Singers on Great Singing*, 5th limelight ed. New York: Limelight Editions, 1990 [Reprint of 1982 ed.].

Hirano, M. *Clinical Examination of Voice*. New York: Springer-Verlag, 1981.

Hixon, Thomas J. *Respiratory Function in Speech and Singing*. Boston: College Hill Press, 1987.

Howell, Peter, Ian Cross, Robert West, eds. *Musical Structure and Cognition*. London: Academic Press, 1985.

Husler, Frederick, and Yvonne Rodd-Marling. *Singing: The Physical Nature of the Vocal Organ*. London: Faber and Faber, 1965.

Joal, Joseph. *On Respiration in Singing*, translated and edited by R. Norris Wolfenden. London: F.J. Rebman, 1895.

Josephs, Jesse J. *The Physics of Musical Sound*. Princeton, N.J.: D. Van Nostrand, 1967.

Judson, Lyman S.V., and Andrew Thomas Weaver. *Voice Science*. New York: Appleton-Century-Crofts, 1942.

Kagen, Sergius. *On Studying Singing*. New York: Dover Publications, 1960.

Kahane, Joel C., and John F. Folkins. *Atlas of Speech and Hearing Anatomy*. Columbus: Charles E. Merrill Publishing, 1984.

Klein, Joseph J., with Ole A. Schjeide. *Singing Technique*. Princeton, N.J.: D. Van Vostrand, 1967.

Ladefoged, Peter. *Elements of Acoustic Phonetics*. Chicago: University of Chicago Press, 1962.

_________. *Three Areas of Experimental Phonetics*. London: Oxford University Press, 1967.

Lamperti, Francesco. *The Art of Singing*, Rev. ed., with translation by J. C. Griffith. New York: G. Schirmer, [1890].

Lankow, Anna. *The Science of the Art of Singing*, 2nd ed. New York: Breitkopf and Haertel, 1902.

Large, John, ed. *Contributions of Voice Research to Singing*. Houston: College-Hill, 1980.

_________. *Vocal Registers in Singing*. The Hague: Mouton, 1973.

Lawrence, Van, ed. *Care of the Professional Voice*, transcripts of the 7th [Part I], 8th, 9th, 10th, 11th, 12th, 13th, and 14th Symposia. New York: Voice Foundation, 1978-1985.

Lehmann, Lilli. *How to Sing*, new rev. and suppl. ed., translated by Richard Aldrich and Clara Willenbuecher. New York: Macmillan, 1952.

Leiser, Clara. *Jean de Reszke and the Great Days of Opera.* Westport, Conn.: Greenwood Press, 1970 [Reprint of 1934 ed.].

Lowery, H. *A Guide to Musical Acoustics.* New York: Dover Publ., 1966 [Reprint of 1956 ed.].

Luchsinger, Richard, and Godfrey E. Arnold. *Voice-Speech-Language.* Belmont, CA: Wadsworth Publishing, 1965.

Mackensie, Morell. *The Hygiene of the Vocal Organs*, 7th ed. New York: Macmillan, 1890.

McKenzie, Duncan. *Training the Boy's Changing Voice.* New Brunswick, N.J.: Rutgers University Press, 1956.

McKinney, James C. *The Diagnosis and Correction of Vocal Faults.* Nashville, TN: Broadman Press, 1982.

Maisel, Edward, comp. *The Resurrection of the Body: The Writings of F. M. Alexander.* New York: Dell Publishing, 1969.

Malmberg, Bertil, ed. *Manual of Phonetics.* Amsterdam: North-Holland Publishing, 1968.

Mancini, Giambattista. *Practical Reflections on Figured Singing*, translated (from the 1774 and 1777 eds.) and edited by Edward Foreman. Champaign, Illinois: Pro Musica Press, 1967.

Manén, Lucie. *The Art of Singing.* London: Faber Music, 1974.

Marafioti, P. Mario. *Caruso's Method of Voice Production.* New York: Dover Publications, 1981 [Reprint of 1922 ed.].

Marchesi, Mathilde. *Ten Singing Lessons.* New York: Harper, 1901.

_________. *Theoretical and Practical Vocal Method.* Reprint ed. New York: Dover Publications, 1970.

Marshall, Madeleine. *The Singer's Manual of English Diction.* New York: G. Schirmer, 1953.

Miller, Richard. *English, French, German and Italian Techniques of Singing.* Metuchen, N.J.: Scarecrow Press, 1977.

_________. *The Structure of Singing.* New York: Schirmer Books, 1986.

Minife, Fred D., Thomas J. Hixon, Frederick Williams, eds. *Normal Aspects of Speech, Hearing, and Language.* Englewood Cliffs, N.J.: Prentice-Hall, 1973.

Monahan, Brent Jeffrey. *The Art of Singing.* Metuchen, N.J.: Scarecrow Press, 1978.

Moses, Paul J. *The Voice of Neurosis.* New York: Grune & Stratton, 1954.

Negus, V.E. *The Comparative Anatomy and Physiology of the Larynx*, 1st ed. London: William Heinemann Medical Books, 1949.

Netter, Frank H. *Atlas of Human Anatomy.* Summit, N.J.: CIBA-GEIGY Corp., 1989.

Olson, Harry F. *Music, Physics and Engineering*, 2nd ed. New York: Dover, 1967.

Paget, Richard. *Human Speech.* New York : AMS Press, 1978 [Reprint of 1930 ed.].

Perkins, William H. and Raymond D. Kent. *Functional Anatomy of Speech, Language and Hearing: A Primer.* Austin, TX: PRO-ED, 1990 [Reprint of 1986 ed.].

Pleasants, Henry. *The Great Singers.* New York: Simon and Schuster, 1966.

Proctor, Donald F. *Breathing, Speech, and Song.* New York: Springer-Verlag, 1980.

Punt, Norman A. *The Singer's and Actor's Throat.* London: William Heinemann Medical Books, 1952.

Redfield, John. *Music.* New York: Tudor Publishing, 1935.

Reid, Cornelius L. *Bel Canto: Principles and Practices.* New York: Patelson Music House, 1978 [Reprint of 1950 ed.].

__________. *The Free Voice.* New York: Coleman-Ross, 1965.

Rose, Arnold. *The Singer and the Voice* [2nd ed.] London: Faber and Faber, 1971.

Rosewall, Richard B. *Handbook of Singing*, Rev. ed. Evanston, Ill.: Dickerson Press, 1984.

Rossing, Thomas. *The Science of Sound.* Reading, Mass.: Addison-Wesley, 1982.

Rushmore, Robert. *The Singing Voice.* New York: Dodd, Mead, 1970.

Sataloff, Robert Thayer. *Professional Voice: The Science and Art of Clinical Care.* New York: Raven Press, 1991.

Sataloff, Robert Thayer, Alice G. Brandfonbrener, Richard J. Lederman, eds. *Textbook of Performing Arts Medicine.* New York: Raven Press, 1991.

Sataloff, Robert T., and Ingo R. Titze, eds. *Vocal Health and Science.* Jacksonville, FL: National Association of Teachers of Singing, 1991.

Saunders, William H., M.D. *The Larynx.* Summit, N.J.: CIBA Pharmaceutical, 1964.

Shakespeare, William. *The Art of Singing.* Bryn Mawr, Pennsylvania: Oliver Ditson, 1921.

__________. *Plain Words on Singing.* Bryn Mawr, Pennsylvania: Oliver Ditson, 1921.

Stanley, Douglas. *The Science of Voice,* 3rd ed. New York: Carl Fischer, 1939.

Stevens, Kenneth N., and Minoru Hirano, eds. *Vocal Fold Physiology.* Tokyo: University of Tokyo Press, 1981.

Sundberg, Johan, ed. *Research Aspects on Singing.* Stockholm: Royal Swedish Academy of Music, 1981.

Sundberg, Johan. *The Science of Musical Sounds.* New York: Academy Press, 1991.

__________. *The Science of the Singing Voice.* DeKalb, IL: Northern Illinois University Press, 1987.

Swanson, Frederick J. *The Male Singing Voice Ages Eight to Eighteen.* Cedar Rapids, Iowa: Laurance Press, 1977.

Taylor, Robert M. *Acoustics for the Singer.* Emporia: Kansas State Teacher's College, 1958.

Titze, Ingo R., and Ronald C. Scherer, eds. *Vocal Fold Physiology: Biomechanics, Acoustics and Phonatory Control.* Denver: Denver Center for the Performing Arts, 1983.

Tosi, Pietro Francesco. *Observations on the Florid Song*, 2nd ed., translated by John Galliard. London: J. Wilcox, 1743.

Uris, Dorothy. *To Sing in English.* New York: Boosey and Hawkes, 1971.

Vaccai, Nicola. *Practical Method of Italian Singing.* Reprint. New York: G. Schirmer, 1975.

Vander, Arthur J., James H. Sherman, Dorothy S. Luciano. *Human Physiology: The Mechanisms of Body Function*, 5th ed. New York: McGraw-Hill, 1990.

Vennard, William. *Singing: The Mechanism and the Technic*, 4th ed. New York: Carl Fischer, 1967.

Wall, Joan. *International Phonetic Alphabet for Singers.* Dallas: PST... Inc., 1988.

Wall, Joan, Robert Caldwell, Tracy Gavilanes, Sheila Allen. *Diction for Singers.* Dallas: PST... Inc., 1990.

Weaver, Andrew Thomas. *Speech: Forms and Principles*, 1st ed. New York: Longmans, Green, 1942.

Weinberg, Bernd, ed. *Care of the Professional Voice, Transcripts of the 7th Symposium Part II.* New York: Voice Foundation, 1978.

Wilson, D. Kenneth. *Voice Problems of Children.* Baltimore: Williams & Wilkins, 1972.

Winckel, Fritz. *Music, Sound and Sensation*, translated by Thomas Binkley. New York: Dover Publications, 1967.

Witherspoon, Herbert. *Singing.* New York: Da Capo Press, 1980 [Reprint of 1925 ed.].

Wood, Alexander. *The Physics of Music*, 6th ed. London: Methuen, 1962.

Wormhoudt, Pearl Shinn. *Building the Voice as an Instrument*. Oskaloosa, IA: William Penn College, 1981.

Young, Gerard Mackworth. *What Happens in Singing*. London: Newman Neame, 1953.

Zemlin, Willard R. *Speech and Hearing Science*. 3rd ed. Englewood Cliffs, N.J.: Prentice-Hall, 1988.

ARTICLES

Abitbol, Jean, Jean de Brux, Ginette Millot, Marie-Francoise Masson, Odile Languille Mimoun, Helene Pau, and Beatrice Abitbol. "Does a Hormonal Cord Cycle Exist in Women?: Study of Vocal Premenstrual Syndrome in Voice Performers by Videostroboscopy-Glottography and Cytology on 38 Women," *Journal of Voice*, 3:2 (1989), 157-162.

Acker, Barbara F., Richard Miller, Bonnie N. Raphael, Lucille S. Rubin, Ronald C. Scherer, and Johan Sundberg [panel]. "The Speaking Voice," *Journal of Voice*, 1:1 (1987), 88-91.

Agren, Karin, and Johan Sundberg. "An Acoustic Comparison of Alto and Tenor Voices," *Journal of Research in Singing*, 1:3 (1978), 26-32.

Alt, David. "Misunderstanding Breath Support for Singers," *Choral Journal*, 30:8 (1990), 33-35.

Atkinson, James E. "Correlation Analysis of the Physiological Factors Controlling Fundamental Voice Frequency," *Journal of the Acoustical Society of America*, 63:1 (1978), 211-222.

Baer, Thomas. "Reflex Activation of Laryngeal Muscles by Sudden Induced Subglottal Pressure Changes," *Journal of the Acoustical Society of America*, 65:5 (1979), 1271-1275.

Baer, Thomas, Fredericka Bell-Berti, and Philip Rubin. "Articulation and Voice Quality," *Care of the Professional Voice*, Transcripts of the Seventh Symposium, Part I, Van Lawrence, ed. New York: Voice Foundation, 1978, 48-53.

Baer, Thomas, J. C. Gore, L. C. Gracco, and P. W. Nye. "Analysis of Vocal Tract Shape and Dimensions Using Magnetic Resonance Imaging: Vowels," *Journal of the Acoustical Society of America*, 90:2, Pt.1 (1991), 799-828.

Baken, R. J., and S. A. Cavallo. "Pre-phonatory Chest Wall Posturing," *Folia Phoniatrica*, 33:4 (1981), 193-203.

Bartholomew, Wilmer T. "The Role of Imagery in Voice Teaching," *MTNA Proceedings*, 1935.

Bastian, Robert. "Hoarseness in Singers," *NATS Bulletin*, 40:3 (1984), 26-27.

Batza, E. M. "Vocal Abuse in the Rock-and-Roll Singer," *Cleveland Clinical Quarterly*, 38 (1971), 35-38.

Benninger, Michael S. "The Whisper and the Whistle: The Role in Vocal Trauma," *Medical Problems of Performing Artists*, 3:4 (1988), 151-154.

Benninger, Michael S., Mark A. Carwell, Eileen M. Finnegan, Richard Miller, and Howard L. Legine. "Flexible Direct Nasopharyngolaryngoscopy in Association with Vocal Pedagogy," *Medical Problems of Performing Artists*, 4:4 (1989), 163-167.

Bishop, Beverly. "Neural Regulation of Abdominal Muscle Contractions," *Sound Production in Man: Annals of the New York Academy of Sciences*, A. Bouhuys, ed. New York: New York Academy of Sciences, 1968, 191-200.

Bless, Diane M., and R. J. Baken. "Assessment of Voice," *Journal of Voice*, 6:2 (1992), 95-97.

Bloothooft, Gerrit, and Reiner Plomp. "The Sound Level of the Singer's Formant in Professional Singing," *Journal of the Acoustical Society of America*, 79:6 (1986), 2028-2033.

_________. "Spectral Analysis of Sung Vowels III. Characteristics of Singers and Modes of Singing," *Journal of the Acoustical Society of America*, 79:3 (1986), 852-864.

Boardman, Susan D. "Singing Styles on Broadway," *NATS Journal*, 46:1 (1989), 4-10, 14, 24.

Bolster, Stephen. "The Fixed Formant Theory and Its Implications for Choral Blend and Choral Diction," *Choral Journal*, 23:6 (1983), 27-33.

Boone, Daniel. "Vocal Hygiene: The Optimal Use of the Larynx," *Journal of Research in Singing*, 4:1 (1980), 35-43.

Bouhuys, A., D. Proctor, J. Mead, and K. H. Stevens. "Pressure-flow Events during Singing," *Annals of New York Academy of Sciences*, 155 (1968), 165-176.

Bradley, Brown. "When Oren Brown and Richard Westenberg Speak ... I Listen!" *Choral Journal*, 25:4 (1984), 17-20.

Brandfonbrener, Alice G. "Beta Blockers in the Treatment of Performance Anxiety," *Medical Problems of Performing Artists*, 5:1 (1990), 23-26.

Bravender, Paul E. "The Effect of Cheerleading on the Female Singing Voice," *NATS Bulletin*, 37:2 (1980), 9-13.

Brewer, David W. "Voice Research: The Next Ten Years," *Journal of Voice*, 3:1 (1989), 7-17.

Brodnitz, Friedrich S. "Hormones and the Singing Voice," *NATS Bulletin*, 28:2 (1971), 16-17.

_________. "On Change of the Voice," *NATS Bulletin*, 40:2 (1983), 24-26.

Brown, W. S., Jr., and Harry Hollien. "Effects of Menstruation on the Singing Voice," *Care of the Professional Voice*, Transcripts of the Twelfth Symposium, Part I, Van Lawrence, ed. New York: Voice Foundation, 1983, 112-116.

Bunch, Meribeth. "A Survey of the Research on Covered and Open Voice Qualities," *NATS Bulletin*, 33:3 (1977), 11-18.

Caire, Jill Bond. "Understanding and Treating Performance Anxiety from a Cognitive-Behavior Therapy Perspective." *NATS Journal*, 47:4 (1991), 27-30. 51.

Calder, Lelia. "The Alexander Work," *NATS Journal*, 42:3 (1986), 19-21.

Carlo, Nicole Scotto di, and Denise Autessere. "Movements of the Velum in Singing," *Journal of Research in Singing*, 11:1 (1987), 3-13.

Carlsson, Gunilla, and Johan Sundberg, "Formant Frequency Tuning in Singing," *Journal of Voice*, 6:3 (1992), 256-260.

Campbell, E. J. Moran. "The Respiratory Muscles," *Sound Production in Man: Annals of the New York Academy of Sciences*, A. Bouhuys, ed. New York: New York Academy of Sciences, 1968, 135-140.

Campbell, William M., and John F. Michel. "The Effects of Auditory Masking on Vocal Vibrato," *Care of the Professional Voice*, Transcripts of the Eighth Symposium, Van Lawrence, ed. New York: Voice Foundation, 1979, 50-55.

Cleveland, Thomas F. "Acoustic Properties of Voice Timbre Types and Their Influence on Voice Classification," *Journal of the Acoustical Society of America*, 61:6 (1977), 1622-1629.

_________. "How to Assist the Singer-Student in Choosing a Voice Health-Care Professional," *NATS Journal*, 47:5 (1991), 30-32.

_________. "Physiological and Acoustical Basis for Vocalises Relating to Subglottal Pressure," *NATS Journal*, 49:2 (1992), 25-26.

Coffin, Berton. "Articulation for Opera, Oratorio, and Recital," *NATS Bulletin*, 32:2 (1976), 26-41.

_________. "The Instrumental Resonance of the Singing Voice," *NATS Bulletin*, 31:2 (1974), 26-39.

_________. "The Relationship of the Breath, Phonation and Resonance in Singing," *NATS Bulletin*, 31:3 (1975), 18-24.

_________. "The Singers Diction," *Historical Vocal Pedagogy Classics*. Metuchen, N.J.: Scarecrow Press, 1989, 282-287.

Coleman, Robert F. "Acoustic and Perceptual Factors in Vibrato," *Care of the Professional Voice*, Transcripts of the Eighth Symposium, Part I, Van Lawrence and B. Weinberg, eds. New York: Voice Foundation, 1979, 36-38.

Coleman, Robert F., Jean Hakes, Douglas M. Hicks, John F. Michel, Lorraine A. Ramig, Howard B. Rothman [panel]. "Discussion on Vibrato," *Journal of Voice*, 1:2 (1987), 168-171.

Collins, Don L. "The Changing Voice--the High School Challenge," *Choral Journal*, 28:3 (1987), 13-17.

Colton, Raymond H. "Glottal Waveform Variations Associated with Different Vocal Intensity Levels," *Care of the Professional Voice*, Transcripts of the Thirteenth Symposium, Part I, Van Lawrence, ed. New York: Voice Foundation, 1984, 39-47.

__________. "Physiological Mechanisms of Vocal Frequency Control: The Role of Tension," *Journal of Voice*, 2:3 (1988), 208-220.

Colton, Raymond H., and Jo Estill. "Perceptual Differentiation of Voice Modes," *Care of the Professional Voice*, Transcripts of the Fifth Symposium. New York: Voice Foundation, 1976.

Cooksey, John M. "The Development of a Contemporary, Eclectic Theory for the Training and Cultivation of the Junior High School Male Changing Voice," *Choral Journal*, 18:2, 3, 4 (1977), 5-14, 5-16, 5-15.

Cooper, Morton. "The Tired Speaking voice and the Negative Effect on the Singing Voice," *NATS Bulletin*, 39:2 (1982), 11-14.

Cornut, Guy and Marc Bouchayer. "Phono-surgery for Singers," *Journal of Voice*, 3:3 (1989), 269-276.

Damste, P.H. "Virilization of Voice Due to Anabolic Steroids," *Folia Phoniatrica*, 16:1 (1964), 10-18.

________. "X-ray Study of Phonation," *Folia Phoniatrica*, 20:2 (1968), 65-88.

Darwin, C. F., and R. B. Gardner. "Mistuning a Harmonic of a Vowel: Grouping and Phase Effects on Vowel Quality," *Journal of the Acoustical Society of America*, 79:3 (1986), 838-845.

Deinse, J.V. van. "On Vocal Registers," *Journal of Research in Singing*, 5:2 (1982), 3-49.

Delattre, Pierre. "Vowel Color and Voice Quality," *NATS Bulletin*, 15:1 (1958), 4-7.

Diercks, Louis. "The Individual in the Choral Situation," *NATS Bulletin*, 17:4 (1961), 6-10.

Doscher, Barbara M. "Breathing: The Motor of the Singing Voice," *Choral Journal*, 27:8 (1987), 17-22.

________. "Exploring the Whys of Intonation Problems," *Choral Journal*, 32:4 (1991), 25-30.

________. "Heads Up!" *Choral Journal*, 24:10 (1984), 5-8.

________. "Teaching Singing," *The Quarterly*, 3:2 (1992), 61-66.

Duarte, Fernando. "The Principles of the Alexander Technique Applied to Singing: The Significance of the 'Preparatory Set'," *Journal of Research in Singing*, 5:1 (December, 1981), 3-21.

Edwin, Robert. "Belting: Once More with Feeling," *NATS Journal*, 46:2 (1989), 29, 46.

_________. "The Language of the Body," *NATS Journal*, 48:4 (1992), 37, 53.

_________. "To Belt or Not to Belt--Maybe is the Answer," *NATS Journal*, 44:3 (1988), 39-40.

_________. "Voice and Speech Dynamics in the Total Personality." *NATS Bulletin*, 38:3 (1982), 38-42.

Emmons, Shirlee. "Breathing for Singing," *Journal of Voice*, 2:1 (1988), 30-35.

Estill, Jo. "Belting and Classic Voice Quality: Some Physiological Differences," *Medical Problems of Performing Artists*, 3:1 (1988), 37-43.

_________. "The Control of Voice Quality," *Care of the Professional Voice*, Transcripts of the Eleventh Symposium, Part II, Van Lawrence, ed. New York: Voice Foundation, 1982, 152-169.

Estill, Jo, Thomas Baer, Kiyoshi Honda, and Katherine S. Harris. "An EMG Study of Supralaryngeal Activity in Six Voice Qualities," *Care of the Professional Voice*, Transcripts of the Twelfth Symposium, Part I, Van Lawrence, ed. New York: Voice Foundation, 1983, 86-91.

_________. "An EMG Study of Supralaryngeal Activity in Six Voice Qualities: Part II," *Care of the Professional Voice*, Transcripts of the Thirteenth Symposium, Part I, Van Lawrence, ed. New York: Voice Foundation, 1984, 65-69.

Evans, Kathryn. "Acoustic Study of Vowel Equalization," *Journal of Research in Singing*, 4:2 (1981), 3-22.

Faaborg-Andersen, Knud, and Aato A. Nonninen. "The Function of the Extrinsic Laryngeal Muscles at Different Pitch Levels," *Acta Otolaryngolica*, 49 (1958), 47.

Fant, Gunnar. "Glottal Flow: Models & Interaction," *Journal of Phonetics*, 14:3/4 (1986), 393-399.

________. "The Relation between Area Functions and the Acoustic Signal," *Phonetica*, 37 (1980), 55-86.

________. "The Voice Source--Theory and Acoustic Modeling," *Vocal Fold Physiology: Biomechanics, Acoustics and Phonatory Control*, Ingo R. Titze and Ronald C. Scherer, eds. Denver: Denver Center for the Performing Arts, 1983, 453-464.

Fant, G., K. Fintoft, J. Liljencrants, B. Lindbloom, and J. Martony. "Formant-Amplitude Measurements," *Journal of Acoustical Society of America*. 25:1 (1963), 1753-1761.

Fant, G., and Q. Lin. "Glottal Voice Source--Vocal Tract Acoustic Interaction," *Quarterly Progress Status Report*, STL-QPSR1. Stockholm: Royal Institute of Technology, 1987, 13-27.

Feder, Robert J. "Coughing and Coughing/Clearing: Normal and Professional Voice Care," *Medical Problems of Performing Artists*, 6:3 (1991), 103-104.

________. "Gargling: Its Efficacy for Laryngeal, Inflammatory, or Edematous Changes," *Medical Problems of Performing Artists*, 4:2 (1989), 97-98.

________. "Vocal Health: A View from the Medical Profession," *Choral Journal*, 30:7 (1990), 23-25.

Fields, Victor A. "Review of the Literature on Vocal Registers," *NATS Bulletin*, 26:3 (1970), 37-39, 53.

Frey, Loryn E. "Temporomandibular Joint Dysfunction in Singers: A Survey," *NATS Journal*, 44:3 (1988), 15-19, 40.

Fritzell, Björn. "Electromyography in the Study of the Velo-Pharyngeal Function," *Folia Phoniatrica*, 31:2 (1979), 93-102.

_________. "Singing and the Health of the Voice," *Research Aspects on Singing*, Johan Sundberg, ed. Stockholm: Royal Swedish Academy of Music, 1981, 97-107.

Fry, D. B. and Lucie Manén. "Basis for Acoustical Study of Singing," *Journal of the Acoustical Society of America*, 29:6 (1957), 690-692.

Gackle, Lynne. "The Adolescent Female Voice: Characteristics of Change and the Stages of Development," *Choral Journal*, 31:8 (1991), 17-25.

Garretson, Robert L. "The Falsettists," *Choral Journal*, 24:1 (1983), 5-7, 9.

Gates, George A., and Phillip J. Montalbo. "The Effect of Low-Dose Beta-Blockade on Performance Anxiety in Singers," *Journal of Voice*, 1:1 (1987), 105-108.

Gauffin, Jan, and Johan Sundberg. "Spectral Correlates of Glottal Voice Source Waveform Characteristics," *Journal of Speech and Hearing Research*, 32:3 (1989), 556-565.

Gay, T., L. J. Boé, and P. Perrier. "Acoustic and Perceptual Effects of Changes in Vocal Tract Constrictions for Vowels," *Journal of the Acoustical Society of America*, 92:3 (1992), 301-1309.

Glaze, Leslie E., Diane M. Bless, and Robin D. Susser. "Acoustic Analysis of Vowel and Loudness Differences in Children's Voices," *Journal of Voice*, 4:1 (1990), 37-44.

Goodwin, Allen W. "An Acoustical Study of Individual Voices in Choral Blend," *Journal of Research in Music Education*, 28:2 (1980), 119-128.

__________. "Resolving Conflicts between Choral Directors and Voice Teachers," *Choral Journal*, 21:1 (1980), 5-7.

Gould, W. J. "Effect of Respiratory and Postural Mechanisms upon Action of the Vocal Cords," *Folia Phoniatrica*, 23:4 (1971), 211-224.

Gould W. J., and Miroshi Okamura. "Respiratory Training of the Singer," *Folia Phoniatrica*, 26:4 (1974), 275-285.

Gramming, Patricia, and Johan Sundberg. "Spectrum Factors Relevant to Phonetogram Measurement," *Journal of the Acoustical Society of America*, 83:6 (1988), 2352-2360.

Grant, Joe. "Improving Pitch and Intonation," *Choral Journal*, 28:5 (1987), 5-9.

Gregg, Jean Westerman. "On Articulation--Part I," *NATS Journal*, 47:5 (1991), 30-32.

__________. "On Support," *NATS Journal*, 47:1 (1990), 38-39.

Guthmiller, John Harold. "The Goals of Vocalizaion: Developing Healthy Voices and the Potential for Expressive Singing," *Choral Journal*, 26:7 (1986), 13-16.

Haapanen, Marja-Leena. "Provoked Laryngeal Dysfunction," *Folia Phoniatrica*, 42:4 (1990), 157-169.

Hanson, Lloyd W. "A Survey of Research on Vocal Falsetto," *NATS Journal*, 43:3 (1987), 9-13.

Harris, Robert L. "The Young Female Voice and Alto," *Choral Journal*, 28:3 (1987), 21-23.

Harris, T. M. "The Pharmacological Treatment of Voice Disorders," *Folia Phoniatrica*, 44:3/4 (1992), 143-154.

Hart, Cecil W., and Jerilyn A. Logemann. "Tonsils and Adenoids and the Professional Musician," *Medical Problems of Performing Artists*, 1:2 (1986), 58-63.

Harvey, Nigel. "Vocal Control in Singing: A Cognitive Approach," *Musical Structure and Cognition*, Peter Howell, Ian Cross, and Robert West, eds. New York: Academic Press, 1985, 287-332.

Hertegard, Stella, Jan Gauffin, and Johan Sundberg. "Open and Covered Singing as Studied by Means of Fiberoptics, Inverse Filtering, and Spectral Analysis," *Journal of Voice*, 4:3 (1990), 220-230.

Hicks, P., and G. J. Troup. "Source Spectrum in Professional Singing," *Folia Phoniatrica*, 32:1 (1980), 23-28.

Higgins, Maureen, and John H. Saxman. "Variations in Vocal Frequency Perturbation across the Menstral Cycle," *Journal of Voice*, 3:3 (1989), 233-243.

Hill, Stan. "Characteristics of Air Flow During Changes in Registration," *NATS Journal*, 43:1 (1986), 16-17.

Hirano, Minoru. "Morphological Structure of the Vocal Cord as a Vibrator and Its Variations," *Folia Phoniatrica*, 26:2 (1974), 89-94.

__________. "Objective Evaluation of the Human Voice: Clinical Aspects," *Folia Phoniatrica*, 41 (1989), 89-144.

Hirano, M., S. Kurita, and T. Kakashima. "The Structure of the Vocal Folds, *Vocal Fold Physiology*, K. N. Stevens and M. Hirano, eds. Tokyo: University of Tokyo Press, 1981, 33-43.

Hirano, Minoru, Shigejiro Kurita, and Shinji Sakaguchi. "Aging of the Vibratory Tissue of Human Vocal Folds," *Acta Otolaryngolica*, 107:5/6 (1989), 428-433.

_________. "Vocal Mechanisms in Singing: Laryngeal and Phoniatric Aspects," *Journal of Voice*, 2:1 (1988), 51-69.

Hirano, M., J. Ohala, and W. Vennard. "The Function of Laryngeal Muscles in Regulating Fundamental Frequency and Intensity of Phonation," *Journal of Speech and Hearing Research*, 12:3 (1969), 616-628.

Hirano, M., W. Vennard, and J. Ohala. "Regulation of Register, Pitch and Intensity of Voice: An Electromyographic Investigation of Intrinsic Laryngeal Muscles," *Folia Phoniatrica*, 22:1 (1970), 1-20.

Hirose, H., and S. Niimi. "The Relationship between Glottal Opening and the Transglottal Pressure Differences during Consonant Production," *Laryngeal Function in Phonation and Respiration*, T. Baer, C. Sasaki, & K. S. Harris, eds. Boston: College-Hill Press, 1987, 381-390.

Hisey, Philip D. "Head Quality versus Nasality: a Review of Some Pertinent Literature," *NATS Bulletin*, 28:2 (1971), 4-15, 18.

Hixon, Thomas J. "Respiratory Function in Speech," *Normal Aspects of Speech, Hearing, and Language*, Fred D. Minifie, Thomas J. Hixon, and Frederick Williams, eds. Englewood Cliffs, NJ: Prentice-Hall, 1971, 73-125.

Hixon, T. J., M. D. Goldman, and J. Mead. "Dynamics of the Chest Wall during Speech Production," *Journal of Speech and Hearing Research*, 19 (1976), 297-356.

Hixon, Thomas J., and Cynthia Hoffman. "Chest Wall Shape in Singing," *Care of the Professional Voice*, Transcripts of the Seventh Symposium, Part I, Van Lawrence, ed. New York: Voice Foundation, 1978, 9-10.

Hollien, Harry. "'Old Voices': What Do We Really Know About Them?" *Journal of Voice*, 1:1 (1987), 2-17.

_________. "Report on Vocal Registers," *Care of the Professional Voice*, Transcripts of the Twelfth Symposium, Part I, Van Lawrence, ed. New York: Voice Foundation, 1983, 1-6.

Hollien, Harry, Gary T. Girard, and Robert F. Coleman. "Vocal Fold Vibratory Patterns of Pulse Register Phonation," *Folia Phoniatrica*, 29:3 (1977), 200-205.

Hollien, Harry, and Elwood Keister. "The Varying Characteristics of the Singer's Formant," *Care of the Professional Voice*, Transcripts of the Seventh Symposium, Part I, Van Lawrence, ed. New York: Voice Foundation, 1978, 40-43.

Hollien, H., and C. Schoenhard. "The Riddle of the 'Middle' Register," *Vocal Fold Physiology: Biomechanics, Acoustics and Phonatory Control*, Ingo R. Titze and Ronald C. Scherer, eds. Denver: Denver Center for the Performing Arts, 1983, 256-269.

Holmberg, Eva B., Robert E. Hillman, Joseph S. Perkell. "Glottal Airflow and Transglottal Air Pressure Measurements for Male and Female Speakers in Soft, Normal, and Loud Voice," *Journal of the Acoustical Society of America*, 84:2 (1988), 511-529.

Holt, Gary A., and Kay Edde Holt. "Medications--Aids to Singing Health?" *NATS Journal*, 45:4 (1989), 21-24.

Honda, Kiyoshi. "Variability Analysis of Laryngeal Muscle Activities," *Vocal Fold Physiology: Biomechanics, Acoustics and Phonatory Control*, Ingo R. Titze and Ronald C. Scherer, eds. Denver: Denver Center for the Performing Arts, 1983, 127-137.

Honda, Kiyoshi, and Osamu Fujimura. "Intrinsic Vowel F^0 and Phrase-final F^0 Lowering: Phonological vs. Biological Explanations," *Vocal Fold Physiology: Acoustic, Perceptual, and Physiological Aspects of Voice Mechanisms*, Jan Gauffin and Britta Hammarberg, eds. San Diego: Singular Publishing Group, 1991, 149-157.

Horii, Yoshiyuki. "Acoustic Analysis of Vocal Vibrato: A Theoretical Interpretation of Data," *Journal of Voice*, 3:1 (1989), 36-43.

________. "Jitter and Shimmer in Sustained Vocal Fry Phonation," *Folia Phoniatrica*, 37 (1985), 81-86.

Horii, Y., and K. Hata. "A Note on Phase Relationships between Frequency and Amplitude Modulations in Vocal Vibrato," *Folia Phoniatrica*, 40:6 (1988), 303-311.

Howell, Peter. "Auditory Feedback of the Voice in Singing," *Vocal Fold Physiology: Biomechanics, Acoustics and Phonatory Control*, Ingo R. Titze and Ronald C. Scherer, eds. Denver: Denver Center for the Performing Arts, 1983, 259-286.

Howie, John, and Pierre Delattre. "An Experimental Study of the Effect of Pitch on the Intelligibility of Vowels," *NATS Bulletin*, 18:4 (1962), 6-9.

Huff-Gackle, Lynne. "The Young Adolescent Female Voice (Ages 11-15): Classification, Placement, and Development of Tone," *Choral Journal*, 25:8 (1985), 15-20.

Isshiki, Nobuhiko. "Vocal Efficiency Index," *Vocal Fold Physiology*, K. N. Stevens and M. Hirano, eds. Tokyo: University of Tokyo Press, 1981, 193-207.

_________. "Vocal Intensity and Air Flow Rate," *Folia Phoniatrica*, 17:2 (1965), 92-104.

Isshiki, Nobuhiko and Robert Ringel. "Air Flow during the Production of Selected Consonants," *Journal of Speech and Hearing Research*, 7:3 (1964), 233-244.

Jackson, M. C. Ametrano. "The High Male Range," *Folia Phoniatrica*, 39:1 (1987), 18-25.

Joiner, James Richard. "The Relationship of the Vocal Folds to Vowel Formation: A Study of Current Research," *Journal of Research in Singing*, 12:1 (1988), 35-41.

Kaiser, James F. "Some Observations on Vocal Tract Operation from a Fluid Flow Point of View," *Vocal Fold Physiology: Biomechanics, Acoustics and Phonatory Control*, Ingo R. Titze and Ronald C. Scherer, eds. Denver: Denver Center for the Performing Arts, 1983, 358-386.

Keidar, Anat, Ingo R. Titze, and Craig Timberlake. "Vibrato Characteristics of Tenors Singing High C's," *Care of the Professional Voice*, Transcripts of the Thirteenth Symposium, Part I, Van Lawrence, ed. New York: Voice Foundation, 1984, 105-110.

Kelman, A. W. "Vibratory Patterns of the Vocal Folds," *Folia Phoniatrica*, 33:2 (1981), 73-99.

Kent, R. D., and A. D. Murray. "Acoustic Features of Infant Vocalic Utterances at 3, 6, and 9 Months," *Journal of the Acoustical Society of America*, 72:2 (1982), 353-365.

Kitzing, Peter. "Photo- and Electroglottographical Recording of the Laryngeal Vibratory Pattern during Different Registers," *Folia Phoniatrica*, 34:5 (1982), 234-241.

Kitzing, Peter, Björn Carlborg, and Anders Löfqvist. "Aerodynamic and Glottographic Studies of the Laryngeal Vibratory Cycle," *Folia Phoniatrica*, 34:4 (1982), 216-224.

Klatt, Dennis H., K. N. Stevens, and J. Mead. "Studies of Articulation Activity and Airflow during Speech," *Sound Production in Man: Annals of the New York Academy of Sciences*, A. Bouhuys, ed. New York: New York Academy of Sciences, 1968, 42-55.

Kmucha, Steven T., Eiji Yanagisawa, and Jo Estill. "Endolaryngeal Changes during High-Intensity Phonation Videolaryngoscopic Observations," *Journal of Voice*, 4:4 (1990), 346-354.

Koizumi, Takuya, Shuji Taniguchi, Seijiro Hiromitsu. "Glottal Source--Vocal Tract Interaction," *Journal of the Acoustical Society of America*, 78:5 (1985), 1541-1547.

Ladefoged, Peter. "Linguistic Aspects of Respiratory Phenomena," *Sound Production in Man: Annals of the New York Academy of Sciences*, A. Bouhuys, ed. New York: New York Academy of Sciences, 1968, 141-151.

Ladefoged, Peter, Richard Harshman, Louis Goldstein, and Loyd Rice. "Generating Vocal Tract Shapes from Formant Frequencies," *Journal of the Acoustical Society of America*, 64:4 (1979), 1027-1035.

Large, John. "Acoustic Study of Register Equalization in Singing," *Folia Phoniatrica*, 25:1 (1973), 39-61.

_________. "Acoustic-Perceptual Evaluation of Register Equalization," *NATS Bulletin*, 31:1 (1974), 20-27, 40-41.

_________. "How to Teach the Male High Voice, Part One: The Tenor," *Journal of Research in Singing*, 9:2 (1986), 3-20.

_________. "How to Teach the Male High Voice, Part Two: The Baritone and Bass," *Journal of Research in Singing*, 10:2 (1987), 17-29.

_________. "Male High Voice Mechanisms in Singing," *Journal of Research in Singing*, 8:1 (1984), 1-10.

_________. "Pedagogy of the Even Scale," *NATS Journal*, 44:2 (1987), 12-16.

_________. "Studies of Extended Vocal Techniques: Safety," *NATS Bulletin*, 34:4 (1978), 30-33.

_________. "Towards an Integrated Physiologic-Acoustic Theory of Vocal Registers," *NATS Bulletin*, 28:3 (1972), 18-36.

Large, John, E. Baird, and T. Jenkins. "Studies of the Male High Voice Mechanisms," *Journal of Research in Singing*, 4:1 (1980), 26-34.

Large, J., and S. Iwata. "Aerodynamic Study of Vibrato and Voluntary 'Strait Tone' Pairs in Singing," *Folia Phoniatrica*, 23:1 (1971), 50-65.

Large, J., S. Iwata, and H. von Leden. "The Male Operatic Head Register versus Falsetto," *Folia Phoniatrica*, 24:1 (1972), 19-29.

________. "The Primary Female Register Transition in Singing," *Folia Phoniatrica*, 22:6 (1970), 385-396.

Large, John, and Thomas Murry. "Studies of the Marchesi Model for Female Registration," *Journal of Research in Singing*, 1:2 (1978), 1-5.

Lawrence, Van. "Cigarettes and Whiskey and Wild, Wild Women," *NATS Bulletin*, 38:3 (1982), 27, 32.

________. "Do Buzzards Roost in Your Mouth at Night?" *NATS Bulletin*, 39:4 (1983), 19-20, 42.

________. "Handy Household Hints: To Sing or Not To Sing," *NATS Bulletin*, 37:3 (1981), 23-25.

________. "Is Allergy Often a Problem for the Singer Who Comes into the Laryngology Office?" *NATS Bulletin*, 40:5 (1984), 20-21, 27.

________. "Laryngological Observations on Belting," *Journal of Research in Singing*, 2:1 (1979), 26-28.

________. "Nodules and Other Things that go Bump in the Night," *NATS Bulletin*, 38:2 (1981), 27, 30.

________. "Nose Drops," *NATS Bulletin*, 39:5 (1983), 26-27.

Lawrence, Van, and Feder, Robert J. "Singing and Flying," *NATS Bulletin*, 41:1 (1984), 26-27.

________. "U.R.I.s," *NATS Bulletin*, 37:4 (1981), 41-42.

________. "What about Cortisone?" *NATS Bulletin*, 38:1 (1981), 28-29.

Leanderson, R., and J. Sundberg. "Breathing for Singing," *Journal of Voice*, 2:1 (1988), 2-12.

Leanderson, R., J. Sundberg, and C. von Euler. "Breathing Muscle Activity and Subglottal Pressure Dynamics in Singing and Speech," *Journal of Voice*, 1:3 (1987), 258-261.

Lennon, John. "'Square One': The Posture of the Body in Singing," *NATS Journal*, 42:2 (1985), 47-50.

Levine, Howard L., and Eileen M. Finnegan. "Overuse and Vocal Disorders: Cause and Effect," *Medical Problems of Performing Artists*, 2:3 (1987), 99-102.

Libin, Barry M., and Michael J. Warren. "Mandibular Posture and the Professional Voice," *NATS Journal*, 44:3 (1988), 11-14.

Lieberman, Philip. "Vocal Cord Motion in Man," *Sound Production in Man: Annals of the New York Academy of Sciences*, A. Bouhuys, ed. New York: New York Academy of Sciences, 1968, 28-41.

Lindblom, Björn, and Johan Sundberg. "Acoustical Consequences of Lip, Tongue, Jaw and Larynx Movements," *Journal of the Acoustical Society of America*, 50:4 (1971), 1166-1179.

Linden, Paul. "Developing Power and Sensitivity through Movement Awareness Training," *American Music Teacher*, 42:2 (1992), 26-31.

Linke, D. E. "A Study of Pitch Characteristics of Female Voices and Their Relationship to Vocal Effectiveness," *Folia Phoniatrica*, 25:3 (1973), 173-185.

Linville, Sue Ellen. "Maximum Phonational Frequency Range Capabilities of Women's Voices with Advancing Age," *Folia Phoniatrica*, 39 (1987), 297-301.

Linville, Sue Ellen, and Hilda B. Fisher. "Acoustic Characteristics of Perceived versus Actual Age in Controlled Phonation by Adult Females," *Journal of the Acoustical Society of America*, 78:1 (1985), 40-48.

Ludlow, Christy L. "Characteristics and Treatment of Laryngeal Dystonias Affecting Voice Users," *Medical Problems of Performing Artists*, 6:4 (1991), 128-131.

McGinnis, C. S., M. Elnick, and M. Kraichman. "A Study of the Vowel Formants of Well-Known Male Operatic Singers," *Journal of the Acoustical Society of America*, 23:4 (1951), 440-446.

McGlone, Robert E., and Marjorie Barstow. "The Effects of the Alexander Technique on Advanced College Singers," *Care of the Professional Voice*, Transcripts of the Seventh Symposium, Part I, Van Lawrence, ed. New York: Voice Foundation, 1978, 66-70.

McGlone, Robert E., and William S. Brown, Jr. "Identification of the 'Shift' between Vocal Registers," *Journal of the Acoustical Society of America*, 46:4, Part 1 (1969), 1033-1036.

McGlone, R.E., and Walter H. Manning. "Role of the Second Formant in Pitch Perception of Whispered and Voiced Vowels," *Folia Phoniatrica*, 31:1 (1979), 9-14.

McGowan, Richard S. "Tongue-tip Trills and Vocal-tract Wall Compliance," *Journal of the Acoustical Society of America*, 91:5 (1992), 2903-2911.

McGowan, R. "An Aeroacoustic Approach to Phonation," *Journal of the Acoustical Society of America*, 83:2 (1988), 696-704.

McHenry, M. A., and A. R. Reich. "Effective Airway Resistance and Vocal Sound Pressure Level in Cheerleaders with a History of Dysphonic Episodes," *Folia Phoniatrica*, 37:5 (1985), 223-231.

McLane, M. "Artistic Vibrato and Tremolo: A Survey of the Literature, Part I," *Journal of Research in Singing*, 8:2 (1985), 21-43.

_________. "Artistic Vibrato and Tremolo: A Survey of the Literature, Part II," *Journal of Research in Singing*, 9:1 (1985), 11-42.

Mabry, Gary. "Head Position and Vocal Production," *Choral Journal*, 33:2 (1992), 31.

Maragos, Nicolas E. "Complications of Endotracheal Intubation in the Singer," *Care of the Professional Voice*, Transcripts of the Tenth Symposium, Van Lawrence, ed. New York: Voice Foundation, 1981, 148-153.

Martensson, A. "The Functional Organization of the Intrinsic Laryngeal Muscles," *Sound Production in Man: Annals of the New York Academy of Sciences*, A. Bouhuys, ed. New York: New York Academy of Sciences, 1968, 91-97.

Martin, F. Gene. "Drugs and Vocal Function," *Journal of Voice*, 2:4 (1988), 338-344.

_________. "Drugs and the Voice," *Care of the Professional Voice*, Transcripts of the Twelfth Symposium, Van Lawrence, ed. New York: Voice Foundation, 1983, 124-132.

_________. "Drugs and the Voice: Part II," *Care of the Professional Voice*, Transcripts of the Eleventh Symposium, Part I, Van Lawrence, ed. New York: Voice Foundation, 1982, 191-201.

Mason, Robert M., and Willard R. Zemlin. "The Phenomenon of Vocal Vibrato," *NATS Bulletin*, 22:3 (1966), 12-17, 37.

Maurer, Dieter, Theodor Landis. "Role of Bone Conduction in the Self-Perception of Speech," *Folia Phoniatrica*, 42:5 (1990), 226-229.

Maxwell, Donald E. "The Effect of White Noise Masking on Singers," *Journal of Research in Singing*, 8:2 (1985), 9-19.

Michel, John F., Robert Coleman, Leslie Guinn, Diane Bless, Craig Timberlake, and Robert T. Sataloff. "Aging Voice: Panel 2," *Journal of Voice*, 1:1 (1987), 62-67.

Michel, John, and John Grashel. "Vocal Vibrato as a Function of Frequency and Intensity," *Care of the Professional Voice*, Transcripts of the Ninth Symposium, Part I, Van Lawrence, ed. New York: Voice Foundation, 1980, 45-48.

Michel, J. F., and R.A. Willis. "An Acoustical Study of Voice Projection," *Care of the Professional Voice*, Transcripts of the Twelfth Symposium, Part I, Van Lawrence, ed. New York: Voice Foundation, 1983, 52-56.

Miles, Beth, and Harry Hollien. "Whither Belting," *Journal of Voice*, 4:1 (1990), 64-70.

Miller, Donald. "Some Observations on the Soprano Voice," *NATS Journal*, 43:5 (1987), 12-15.

Miller, Richard. "Diction and Vocal Technique," *NATS Bulletin*, 38:3 (1982), 43.

_________. "Imagery and the Teaching of Singing," *NATS Journal*, 46:1 (1989), 15-16.

_________. "Supraglottal Considerations and Vocal Pedagogy," *Care of the Professional Voice*, Transcripts of the Ninth Symposium, Part II, Van Lawrence, ed. New York: Voice Foundation, 1980, 55-63.

_________. "Taming the Terrible Triplets: Tongue/Hyoid Bone/Larynx," *NATS Journal*, 43:5 (1987), 33-35, 42.

_________. "Vibrato in Relation to the Vocal Legato." *NATS Bulletin*, 22:3 (1966), 10-21.

Miller, Richard, and Erkki Bianco. "Diaphragmatic Action in Three Approaches to Breath Management in Singing," *Care of the Professional Voice*, Transcripts of the Fourteenth Symposium, Part I, Van Lawrence, ed. New York: Voice Foundation, 1985, 357-360.

Miller, Richard, and Juan Carlos Franco. "A Brief Spectral Study of Vowel Differentiation and Modification in a Professional Tenor Voice," *NATS Journal*, 49:2 (1992), 7-9.

Miller, Richard, and Harm K. Schutte. "The Effect of Tongue Position on Spectra in Singing," *NATS Bulletin*, 37:3 (1981), 26-27, 34.

Milutinovic, Zoran. "Results of Vocal Therapy for Phononeurosis: Behavior Approach," *Folia Phoniatrica*, 42:4 (1990), 173-177.

Milutinovic, Z., M. Sastovka, M. Vohradnik, S. Janosevic. "EMG Study of Hyperkinetic Phonation Using Surface Electrodes," *Folia Phoniatrica*, 40:1 (1988), 21-30.

Moore, Paul, and Hans von Leden. "Dynamic Variations of the Vibratory Pattern in the Normal Larynx," *Folia Phoniatrica*, 10 (1958), 205-238.

Morris, Richard J., and W. S. Brown, Jr. "Age-Related Voice Measures Among Adult Women," *Journal of Voice*, 1:1 (1987), 38-43.

Morrish, Kathleen A., Maureen Stone, Thomas H. Shawker, and Barbara C. Sonies. "Distinguishability of Tongue Shape during Vowel Production," *Journal of Phonetics*, 13:2 (1985), 189-203.

Murray, Alexander. "The Alexander Technique," *Medical Problems of Performing Artists*, 1:4 (1986), 131-132.

Murry, Thomas, and W. S. Brown, Jr. "Aerodynamic Interactions Associated with Voiced-Voiceless Stop Consonants," *Folia Phoniatrica*, 31:1 (1979), 82-88.

Murry, Thomas, and Gayle E. Woodson. "A Comparison of Three Methods for the Management of Vocal Fold Nodules," *Journal of Voice*, 6:3 (1992), 271-276.

Myers, Denise, and John Michel. "Vibrato and Pitch Transitions," *Journal of Voice*, 1:2 (1987), 157-161.

Nelson, Howard D., and William R. Tiffany. "The Intelligibility of Song," *NATS Bulletin*, 25:2 (1968), 22-28.

Nies, Alan S. "Clinical Pharmacology of Beta-Adrenergic Blockers," *Medical Problems of Performing Artists*, 5:1 (1990), 27-32.

Nimii, Seiji, Fredericka Bell-Berti, and Katherine S. Harris. "Dynamic Aspects of Velopharyngeal Closure," *Folia Phoniatrica*, 34 (1982), 246-257.

Nubé, Jacqueline. "Beta-Blockers: Effects on Performing Musicians," *Medical Problems of Performing Artists*, 6:2 (1991), 61-68.

Ocker, Claus, Wolfgang Pascher, Marianne Röhrs, and Walburg Katny. "Voice Disorders Among Players of Wind Instruments," *Folia Phoniatrica*, 42:1 (1990), 24-30.

Oncley, Paul. "Acoustics of the Singing Voice," *Journal of the Acoustical Society of America*, 26:5 (1953), 932.

_________. "Frequency Amplitude and Waveform Modulation in the Vocal Vibrato," *Journal of the Acoustical Society of America*, 49 (1971), 132.

Osborne, Conrad. "The Broadway Voice. Part I: Just Singing in the Pain," *High Fidelity*, 29:1 (1979a), 57-65.

_________. "The Broadway Voice. Part II: Just Singing in the Pain," *High Fidelity*, 29:1 (1979b), 53-56.

Perkins, William H. "Mechanisms of Vocal Abuse," *Care of the Professional Voice*, Transcripts of the Seventh Symposium, Van Lawrence, ed. New York: Voice Foundation, 1978, 106-115.

Pershall, Kim E., and Daniel R. Boone. "Supra-Glottic Contribution to Voice Quality," *Journal of Voice*, 1:2 (1987), 186-190.

Pesak, Josef. "Complex Mechanism of Laryngeal Phonation: A Description of Activity," *Folia Phoniatrica*, 42:4 (1990), 201-207.

_________. "Complex Mechanism of Laryngeal Phonation: Analogue Pattern of the Larynx," *Folia Phoniatrica*, 42:4 (1990), 208-212.

Peterson, Gordon E., and Harold L. Barney. "Control Methods Used in a Study of the Vowels," *Journal of the Acoustical Society of America*, 24:2 (1952), 175-184.

Peterson, Gordon E., and J. E. Shoup. "The Elements of an Acoustic Phonetic Theory," *Journal of Speech and Hearing Research*, 9 (1966), 68-99.

Photiadis, Douglas M. "The Effect of Wall Elasticity on the Properties of a Helmholtz Resonator," *Journal of the Acoustical Society of America*, 90:2, pt.1 (1991), 1188-1190.

Proctor, Donald F. "Breath, the Power Source of the Voice," *NATS Bulletin*, 37:2 (1980), 26-30.

_________. "The Physiologic Basis of Voice Training," *Sound Production in Man: Annals of the New York Academy of Sciences*, A. Bouhuys, ed. New York: New York Academy of Sciences, 1968, 208-228.

Raphael, Bonnie. "Improving the Singer's Speaking Voice," *NATS Journal*, 43:2 (1986), 9-13.

Read, Donald, and Clifford Osborne. "The Three Variables, the Break and Registration," *NATS Bulletin*, 37:5 (1981), 19-20.

Reid, Cornelius L. "The Nature of Vibrato," *Journal of Research in Singing*, 12:2 (1989), 39-61.

Reinders, Ank. "Falsetto Usage, Past and Present," *NATS Journal*, 42:1 (1985), 12-15.

_________. "Teaching the High Female Voice," *Journal of Research in Singing*, 12:1 (1988), 43-46.

Ringel, Robert L., and Wojtek J. Chodzko-Zajko. "Vocal Indices of Biological Age," *Journal of Voice*, 1:1 (1987), 31-37.

Roch, J. B., F. Comte, A. Eyraud, C. Dubreuil. "Synchronization of Glottography and Laryngeal Stroboscopy," *Folia Phoniatrica*, 42:6 (1990), 289-295.

Rossing, Thomas D., Johan Sundberg, and Sten Ternström. "Acoustic Comparison of Soprano Solo and Choir

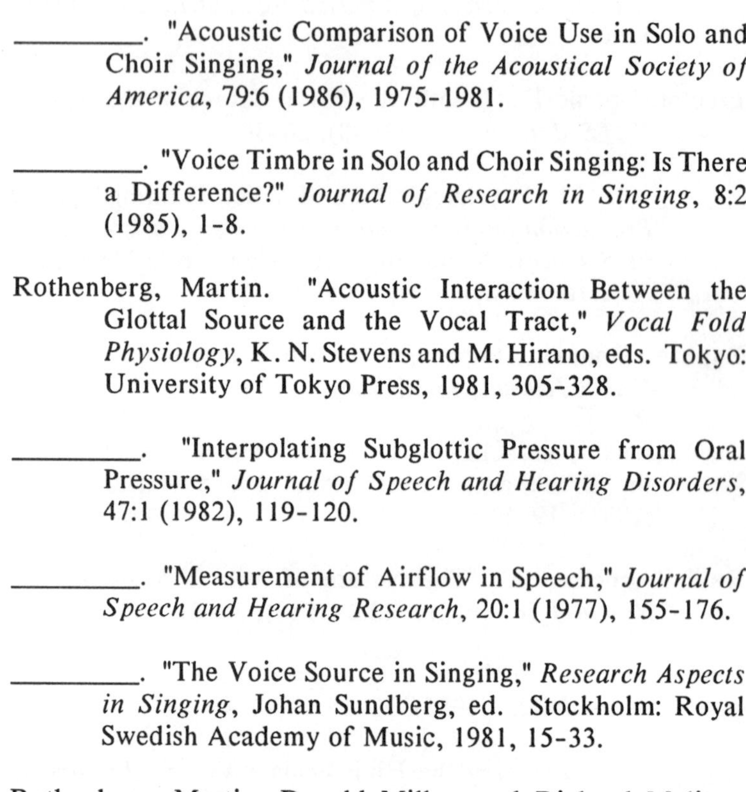

Singing," *Journal of the Acoustical Society of America*, 82:3 (1987), 830-836.

_________. "Acoustic Comparison of Voice Use in Solo and Choir Singing," *Journal of the Acoustical Society of America*, 79:6 (1986), 1975-1981.

_________. "Voice Timbre in Solo and Choir Singing: Is There a Difference?" *Journal of Research in Singing*, 8:2 (1985), 1-8.

Rothenberg, Martin. "Acoustic Interaction Between the Glottal Source and the Vocal Tract," *Vocal Fold Physiology*, K. N. Stevens and M. Hirano, eds. Tokyo: University of Tokyo Press, 1981, 305-328.

_________. "Interpolating Subglottic Pressure from Oral Pressure," *Journal of Speech and Hearing Disorders*, 47:1 (1982), 119-120.

_________. "Measurement of Airflow in Speech," *Journal of Speech and Hearing Research*, 20:1 (1977), 155-176.

_________. "The Voice Source in Singing," *Research Aspects in Singing*, Johan Sundberg, ed. Stockholm: Royal Swedish Academy of Music, 1981, 15-33.

Rothenberg, Martin, Donald Miller, and Richard Molitor. "Aerodynamic Investigation of Sources of Vibrato," *Folia Phoniatrica*, 40:5 (1988), 244-260.

Rothenberg, Martin, and Karen Nezelek. "Airflow-based Analysis of Vocal Function," *Vocal Fold Physiology: Acoustic, Perceptual, and Physiological Aspects of Voice Mechanisms*, Jan Gauffin and Britta Hammarberg, eds. San Diego: Singular Publishing Group, 1991, 139-148.

Rothman, Howard. "Vibrato, What is it?" *NATS Journal*, 43:4 (1987), 16-19.

Roubeau, B., C. Chevrie-Muller, C. Arabia-Guidet. "Electroglottographic Study of the Changes of Voice Registers," *Folia Phoniatrica*, 39 (1987), 280-289.

Rubin, Henry J. "Role of the Laryngologist in Management of Dysfunctions of the Singing Voice," *NATS Bulletin*, 22:4 (1966), 22-27.

Rubin, Henry J., and Charles C. Hirt. "The Falsetto: A High Speed Cinematographic Study," *Laryngoscope*, 70 (1960), 1305-1324.

Rubin, Henry J., M. LeCover, and W. Vennard. "Vocal Intensity, Subglottic Pressure and Air Flow Relationships in Singers," *Folia Phoniatrica*, 19:6 (1967), 393-413.

Ruhl, Jacqueline. "Is Singing a Dying Art?" *NATS Journal*, 42:3 (1986), 30-35.

Russo, Vincent, and John Large. "Psychoacoustic Study of the Bel Canto Model for Register Equalization: Male Chest and Falsetto," *Journal of Research in Singing*, 2:1 (1978), 1-25.

Rutkowski, Joanne. "The Junior High School Male Changing Voice: Testing and Grouping Voices for Successful Singing Experiences," *Choral Journal*, 22:4 (1981), 11-15.

Sallström, Gunvar M., and Jan F. Sallström. "On Training the Singing Voice," *NATS Bulletin*, 34:2 (1977), 18-24.

Sataloff, Robert T. "Common Diagnoses and Treatments in Professional Voice Users," *Medical Problems of Performing Artists*, 2:1 (1987), 15-20.

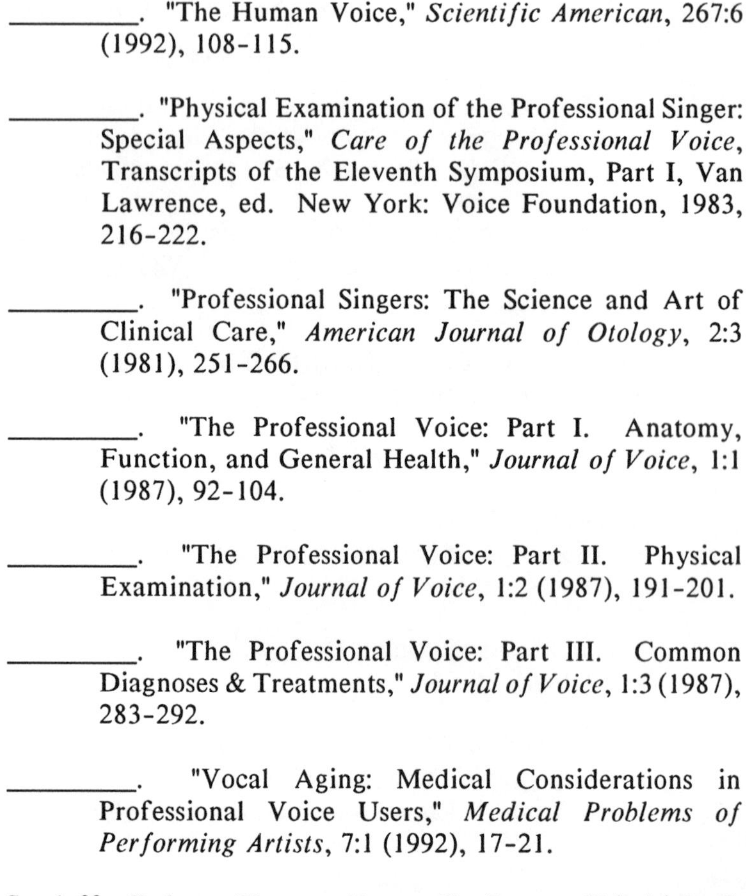

_________. "The Human Voice," *Scientific American*, 267:6 (1992), 108-115.

_________. "Physical Examination of the Professional Singer: Special Aspects," *Care of the Professional Voice*, Transcripts of the Eleventh Symposium, Part I, Van Lawrence, ed. New York: Voice Foundation, 1983, 216-222.

_________. "Professional Singers: The Science and Art of Clinical Care," *American Journal of Otology*, 2:3 (1981), 251-266.

_________. "The Professional Voice: Part I. Anatomy, Function, and General Health," *Journal of Voice*, 1:1 (1987), 92-104.

_________. "The Professional Voice: Part II. Physical Examination," *Journal of Voice*, 1:2 (1987), 191-201.

_________. "The Professional Voice: Part III. Common Diagnoses & Treatments," *Journal of Voice*, 1:3 (1987), 283-292.

_________. "Vocal Aging: Medical Considerations in Professional Voice Users," *Medical Problems of Performing Artists*, 7:1 (1992), 17-21.

Sataloff, Robert Thayer, Barry C. Baron, Friedrich S. Brodnitz, Van L. Lawrence, Wallace Rubin, Joseph Spiegel, and Gayle Woodson [panel]. "Acute Medical Problems of the Voice," *Journal of Voice*, 2:4 (1988), 345-353.

Sataloff, Robert Thayer, Donald O. Castell, Alyson Jones, and Joseph R. Spiegel. "Gastroesophageal Reflux Laryngitis," *NATS Journal*, 49:2 (1992), 21-22.

Sataloff, Robert T., and Joseph R. Spiegel. "Objective Evaluation of the Voice," *Medical Problems of Performing Artists*, 3:3 (1988), 105-108.

________. "The Young Voice," *NATS Journal*, 45:3 (1989), 35-37.

Sawashima, M., S. Niimi, S. Horiguchi, H. Yamaguchi. "Expiratory Lung Pressure, Airflow Rate, and Vocal Intensity: Data on Normal Subjects," *Vocal Fold Physiology: Voice Productions, Mechanisms and Functions*, O. Fujimura, ed. New York: Raven Press, 1988, 415-422.

Scherer, Ronald C., and Ingo R. Titze. "A New Look at Van den Berg's Glottal Aerodynamics," *Care of the Professional Voice*, Transcripts of the Tenth Symposium, Part I, Van Lawrence, ed. New York: Voice Foundation, 1981, 74-81.

Schiff, Maurice, and Wilbur J. Gould. "Hormones and Their Influence on the Performer's Voice," *Care of the Professional Voice*, Transcripts of the Seventh Symposium, Part III, Van Lawrence, ed. New York: Voice Foundation, 1978, 43-48.

Schoenhard, Carol, and Harry Hollien. "A Perceptual Study of Registration in Female Singers," *NATS Bulletin*, 39:1 (1982), 22-26.

Schoenhard, Carol, Harry Hollien, and James W. Hicks, Jr. "Spectral Characteristics of Voice Registers in Female Singers." *Care of the Professional Voice*, Transcripts of the Twelfth Symposium, Part I, Van Lawrence, ed. New York: Voice Foundation, 1983, 7-11.

Schutte, H. K. "Aerodynamics of Phonation," *Acta Oto-Rhino-Laryngol. Belg.*, 40 (1986), 344-357.

________. "Efficiency of Professional Singing Voices in Terms of Energy Ratio," *Folia Phoniatrica*, 36:6 (1984), 267-272.

Schutte, H. K., and R. Miller. "Intra-individual Parameters of the Singer's Formant," *Folia Phoniatrica*, 37:2 (1985), 31-35.

__________. "Resonance Balance in Register Categories of the Singing Voice: A Spectral Analysis Study," *Folia Phoniatrica*, 36:6 (1984), 289-295.

Sears, T., and J. Newsom Davis. "The Control of Respiratory Muscles during Voluntary Breathing," *Sound Production in Man: Annals of the New York Academy of Sciences*, A. Bouhuys, ed. New York: New York Academy of Sciences, 1968, 183-190.

Sells, Michael. "Modern Vocal Pedagogy: An Alternative," *NATS Bulletin*, 27:1 (1970), 35, 50.

Shipp, Thomas. "Vertical Laryngeal Position in Singing," *Journal of Research in Singing*, 1:1 (1977), 16-24.

__________. "Vertical Laryngeal Position: Research Findings & Application for Singers," *Journal of Voice*, 1:3 (1987), 217-219.

Shipp, Thomas, E. Thomas Doherty, and Stig Haglund. "Physiologic Factors in Vocal Vibrato Production," *Journal of Voice*, 4:4 (1990), 300-304.

Shipp, Thomas, Rolf Leanderson, and Stig Haglund. "Contributions of the Crico-thyroid Muscle to Vocal Vibrato," *Care of the Professional Voice*, Transcripts of the Eleventh Symposium, Part I, Van Lawrence, ed. New York: Voice Foundation, 1982, 131-133.

Shipp, Thomas, Per-Aka Lindestad, Frances Mac Curtain, John S. Walker, and Graham F. Welch. "Whistle Register and Falsetto Voice [Panel]," *Journal of Voice*, 2:2 (1988), 164-167.

Shipp, Thomas, and Robert E. McGlone. "Laryngeal Dynamics Associated with Voice Frequency Change," *Journal of Speech and Hearing Research*, 14:4 (1971), 761-768.

Shipp, Thomas, and Philip Morrissey. "Physiologic Adjustments for Frequency Change in Trained and Untrained Voices," *Journal of the Acoustical Society of America*, 62:2 (1977), 476-478.

__________. "Rate and Extent of Vibrato as a Function of Vowel, Effort and Frequency," *Care of the Professional Voice*, Transcripts of the Eighth Symposium, Van Lawrence, ed. New York: Voice Foundation, 1979, 46-49.

Shipp, Thomas, Johan Sundberg, and E. Thomas Doherty. "The Effect of Delayed Auditory Feedback on Vocal Vibrato," *Journal of Voice*, 2:3 (1988), 195-199.

Slawson, W. W. "Vowel Quality and Musical Timbre as Functions of Spectrum Envelope and Fundamental Frequency," *Journal of Acoustical Society of America*, 43:1 (1968), 87-101.

Small, Arnold M. "Acoustics," *Normal Aspects of Speech, Hearing, and Language*, Fred D. Minifie, Thomas J. Hixon, and Frederick Williams, eds. Englewood Cliffs, NJ: Prentice-Hall, 1973, 343-420.

Smith, Lloyd A., and Brian L. Scott. "Increasing the Intelligibility of Sung Vowels," *Journal of the Acoustical Society of America*, 67:5 (1980), 1795-1797.

Sonninen, Aato A. "The External Frame Function in the Control of Pitch in the Human Voice," *Sound Production in Man: Annals of the New York Academy of Sciences*, A. Bouhuys, ed. New York: New York Academy of Sciences, 1968, 68-90.

_________. "Is the Length of the Vocal Cords the Same at All Different Levels of Singing?" *Acta Otolaryngolica*, supplement 118 (1954), 219.

Sonninen, A., P. H. Damste, J. Jol, and J. Fokkens. "On Vocal Strain," *Folia Phoniatrica*, 24:5 (1972), 321-336.

Spencer, Linda E. "Imagery and Anatomy," *NATS Journal*, 46:2 (1989), 28.

Stevens, Kenneth, and A. S. Hours. "Perturbation of Vowel Articulations by Consonantal Context: An Acoustical Study," *Journal of Speech and Hearing Research*, 6:1 (1963), 111-128.

Stone, Maureen, Kathleen A. Morrish, Barbara C. Sonies, and Thomas H. Shawker. "Tongue Curvature: A Model of Shape during Vowel Production," *Folia Phoniatrica*, 39:6 (1987), 302-315.

_________. "Vocal Ligaments Versus Registers," *NATS Bulletin*, 20:2 (1963), 16-21, 31.

Strong, M. Stuart. "Work-related Injuries of Professional Singers: Their Significance and Management," *Vocal Fold Physiology: Voice Productions, Mechanisms and Functions*, O. Fujimura, ed. New York: Raven Press, 1988, 459-464.

Sullivan, Jan. "How to Teach the Belt/Pop Voice," *Journal of Research in Singing*, 13:1 (1989), 41-58.

Sundberg, Johan. "Acoustical Interpretation of the Singers' Formant," *Journal of the Acoustical Society of America*, 55 (1974), 838-844.

_________. "The Acoustics of the Singing Voice," *Scientific American*, 236:3 (March, 1977), 82-91.

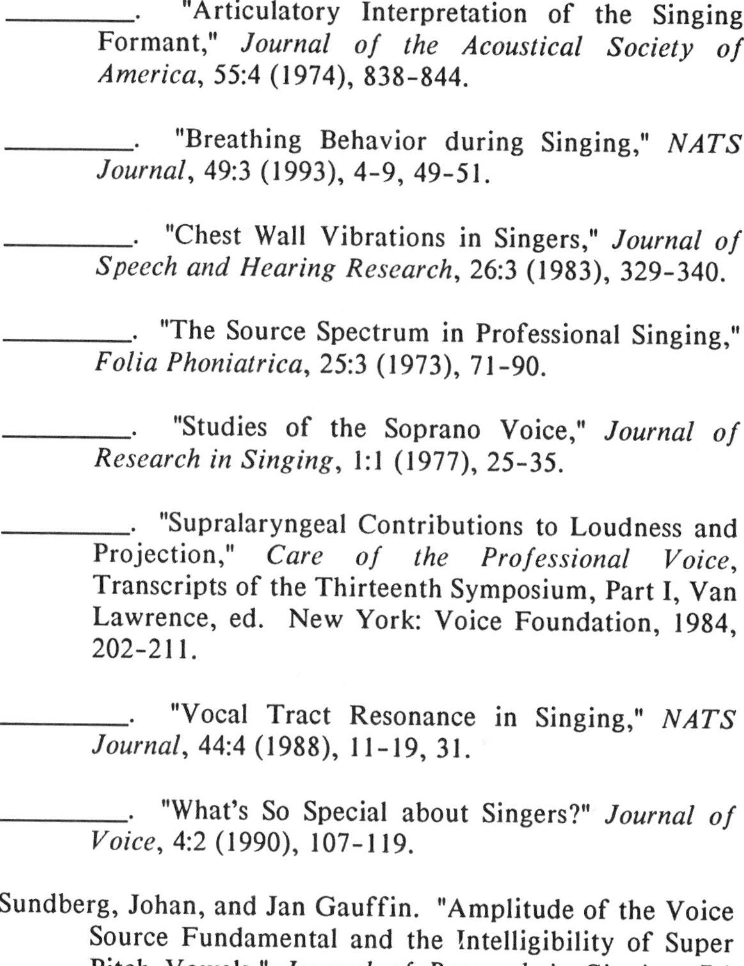

_________. "Articulatory Interpretation of the Singing Formant," *Journal of the Acoustical Society of America*, 55:4 (1974), 838-844.

_________. "Breathing Behavior during Singing," *NATS Journal*, 49:3 (1993), 4-9, 49-51.

_________. "Chest Wall Vibrations in Singers," *Journal of Speech and Hearing Research*, 26:3 (1983), 329-340.

_________. "The Source Spectrum in Professional Singing," *Folia Phoniatrica*, 25:3 (1973), 71-90.

_________. "Studies of the Soprano Voice," *Journal of Research in Singing*, 1:1 (1977), 25-35.

_________. "Supralaryngeal Contributions to Loudness and Projection," *Care of the Professional Voice*, Transcripts of the Thirteenth Symposium, Part I, Van Lawrence, ed. New York: Voice Foundation, 1984, 202-211.

_________. "Vocal Tract Resonance in Singing," *NATS Journal*, 44:4 (1988), 11-19, 31.

_________. "What's So Special about Singers?" *Journal of Voice*, 4:2 (1990), 107-119.

Sundberg, Johan, and Jan Gauffin. "Amplitude of the Voice Source Fundamental and the Intelligibility of Super Pitch Vowels," *Journal of Research in Singing*, 7:1 (1983), 1-5.

Sundberg, Johan, and Rolf Leanderson, "Phonatory Breathing--Physiology Behind Voice Pedagogy: A Tutorial," *Journal of Research in Singing*, 10:1 (1986), 3-21.

Sundberg, Johan, Rolf Leanderson, and Curt von Euler. "Voice Source Effects of Diaphragmatic Activity in Singing," *Journal of Phonetics*, 14:3/4 (1986), 351-357.

Sundberg, Johan, Björn Lindblom, Johan Liljencrants. "Formant Frequency Estimates for Abruptly Changing Area Functions: A Comparison Between Calculations and Measurements," *Journal of the Acoustical Society of America*, 91:6 (1992), 3478-3482.

Sundberg, Johan, and P. E. Nordstrom. "Raised and Lowered Larynx: the Effect on Vowel Formant Frequencies," *Journal of Research in Singing*, 6:2 (1983), 7-15.

Sundberg, J., and M. Rothenberg. "Some Phonatory Characteristics of Singers and Non-Singers," *Quarterly Progress Status Report*, STL-QPSR4, Dept. of Speech Communication and Music Acoustics. Stockholm: Royal Institute of Technology.

Swanson, Frederick J. "The Countertenor in the Last Two Decades of the Twentieth Century," *Choral Journal*, 29:2 (1988), 23-27.

Swing, Dolf. "Teaching the Professional Broadway Voice," *NATS Bulletin*, 29:3 (1973), 38-41.

Taff, Merle E. "An Acoustic Study of Vowel Modification and Register Transition in the Male Singing Voice," *NATS Bulletin*, 22:2 (1965), 5-11, 35.

Tanaka, Shinzo, and Masahiro Tanabe. "Experimental Study on Regulation of Vocal Pitch," *Journal of Voice*, 3:2 (1989), 93-98.

Teachey, Jerold C., Joel C. Kahane, and Neal S. Beckford. "Vocal Mechanics in Untrained Professional Singers," *Journal of Voice*, 5:1 (1991), 51-56.

Ternström, Sten. "Physical and Acoustic Factors that Interact with the Singer to Produce the Choral Sound," *Journal of Voice*, 5:2 (1991), 128-143.

Ternström, Sten, and Johan Sundberg. "Acoustical Aspects of Choir Singing," *Care of the Professional Voice*, Transcripts of the Thirteenth Symposium, Part I, Van Lawrence, ed. New York: Voice Foundation, 1984, 48-52.

_________. "Intonation Precision of Choir Singers," *Journal of the Acoustical Society of America*, 84:1 (1988), 59-69.

Thurman, Leon. "Voice Education in School Music Education," *Care of the Professional Voice*, Transcripts of the Thirteenth Symposium, Part II, Van Lawrence, ed. New York: Voice Foundation, 1984, 455-459.

_________. "Voice Health and Choral Singing: When Voice Classifications Limit Singing Ability," *Choral Journal*, 28:10 (1988), 25-33.

Thurman, Leon, and Van Lawrence. "Voice Care for Vocal Athletes in Training," *The Choral Journal*, 20:9 (1980), 34-37, 56.

Timberlake, Craig. "Loudness and Projection as Related to Vocal Pedagogy," *Care of the Professional Voice*, Transcripts of the Thirteenth Symposium, Part I, Van Lawrence, ed. New York: Voice Foundation, 1984, 245-254.

_________. "Terminological Turmoil--the Naming of Registers," *NATS Journal*, 47:1 (1990), 24-26.

Titze, Ingo R. "A Brief Introduction to Muscles," *NATS Journal*, 46:4 (1990), 16, 21.

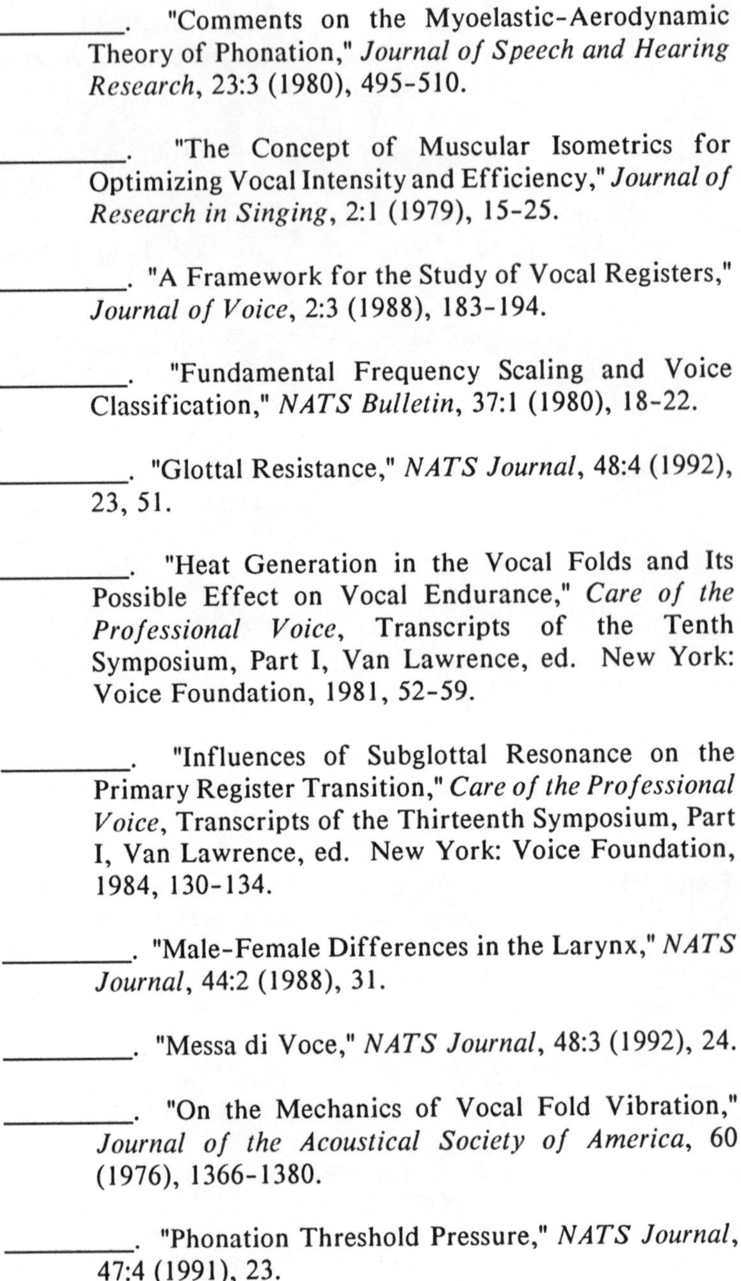

_________. "Comments on the Myoelastic-Aerodynamic Theory of Phonation," *Journal of Speech and Hearing Research*, 23:3 (1980), 495-510.

_________. "The Concept of Muscular Isometrics for Optimizing Vocal Intensity and Efficiency," *Journal of Research in Singing*, 2:1 (1979), 15-25.

_________. "A Framework for the Study of Vocal Registers," *Journal of Voice*, 2:3 (1988), 183-194.

_________. "Fundamental Frequency Scaling and Voice Classification," *NATS Bulletin*, 37:1 (1980), 18-22.

_________. "Glottal Resistance," *NATS Journal*, 48:4 (1992), 23, 51.

_________. "Heat Generation in the Vocal Folds and Its Possible Effect on Vocal Endurance," *Care of the Professional Voice*, Transcripts of the Tenth Symposium, Part I, Van Lawrence, ed. New York: Voice Foundation, 1981, 52-59.

_________. "Influences of Subglottal Resonance on the Primary Register Transition," *Care of the Professional Voice*, Transcripts of the Thirteenth Symposium, Part I, Van Lawrence, ed. New York: Voice Foundation, 1984, 130-134.

_________. "Male-Female Differences in the Larynx," *NATS Journal*, 44:2 (1988), 31.

_________. "Messa di Voce," *NATS Journal*, 48:3 (1992), 24.

_________. "On the Mechanics of Vocal Fold Vibration," *Journal of the Acoustical Society of America*, 60 (1976), 1366-1380.

_________. "Phonation Threshold Pressure," *NATS Journal*, 47:4 (1991), 23.

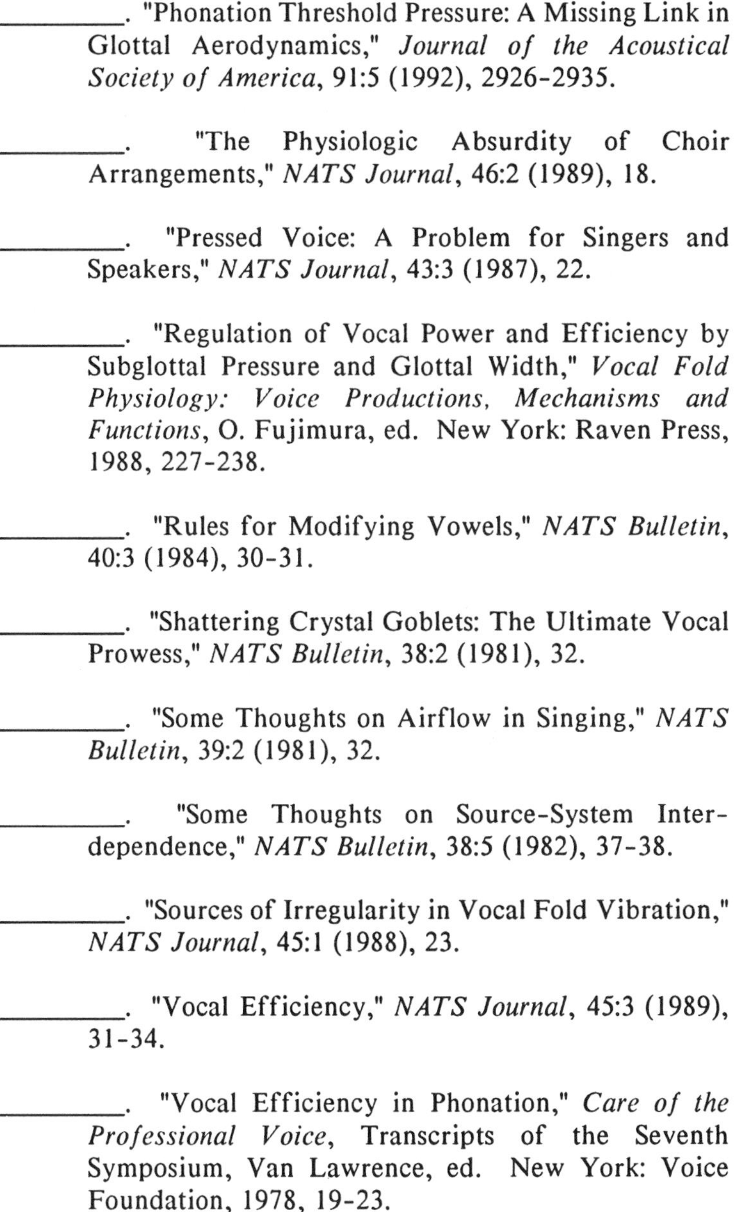

_________. "Phonation Threshold Pressure: A Missing Link in Glottal Aerodynamics," *Journal of the Acoustical Society of America*, 91:5 (1992), 2926-2935.

_________. "The Physiologic Absurdity of Choir Arrangements," *NATS Journal*, 46:2 (1989), 18.

_________. "Pressed Voice: A Problem for Singers and Speakers," *NATS Journal*, 43:3 (1987), 22.

_________. "Regulation of Vocal Power and Efficiency by Subglottal Pressure and Glottal Width," *Vocal Fold Physiology: Voice Productions, Mechanisms and Functions*, O. Fujimura, ed. New York: Raven Press, 1988, 227-238.

_________. "Rules for Modifying Vowels," *NATS Bulletin*, 40:3 (1984), 30-31.

_________. "Shattering Crystal Goblets: The Ultimate Vocal Prowess," *NATS Bulletin*, 38:2 (1981), 32.

_________. "Some Thoughts on Airflow in Singing," *NATS Bulletin*, 39:2 (1981), 32.

_________. "Some Thoughts on Source-System Interdependence," *NATS Bulletin*, 38:5 (1982), 37-38.

_________. "Sources of Irregularity in Vocal Fold Vibration," *NATS Journal*, 45:1 (1988), 23.

_________. "Vocal Efficiency," *NATS Journal*, 45:3 (1989), 31-34.

_________. "Vocal Efficiency in Phonation," *Care of the Professional Voice*, Transcripts of the Seventh Symposium, Van Lawrence, ed. New York: Voice Foundation, 1978, 19-23.

________. "Vocal Registers," *NATS Bulletin*, 39:4 (1983), 21-22, 27.

________. "What Determines the Elastic Properties of the Vocal Folds and How Important are They?" *NATS Bulletin*, 38:1 (1981), 30-31.

________. "Why is the Verbal Message Less Intelligible in Singing than in Speech?" *NATS Bulletin*, 38:3 (1982), 37.

________. "A Word about Words," *NATS Journal*, 45:4 (1989), 19-20.

Titze, Ingo, and W. J. Strong. "Simulated Vocal Cord Motions in Speech and Singing." *Journal of the Acoustical Society of America*, 52:1 (1972), 123-124.

Titze, Ingo R., and Johan Sundberg. "Vocal Intensity in Speakers and Singers," *Journal of the Acoustical Society of America*, 91:5 (1992), 2936-2946.

Titze, Ingo, and David T. Talkin. "A Theoretical Study of the Effects of Various Laryngeal Configurations on the Acoustics of Phonation," *Journal of the Acoustical Society of America*, 66:1 (1979), 60-74.

Troup, G. J., G. Welch, M. Volo, A. Tronconi, F. Ferrero, and E. Farnetani. "On Velum Opening in Singing," *Journal of Research in Singing*, 13:1 (1989), 35-39.

Van Deinse, J. B. "Registers," *Folia Phoniatrica*, 33:1 (1981), 37-50.

Van den Berg, Janwillem. "Mechanism of the Larynx and the Laryngeal Vibrations," *Manual of Phonetics*, Bertil Malmberg, ed. Amsterdam: North-Holland Publishing, 1968, 278-308.

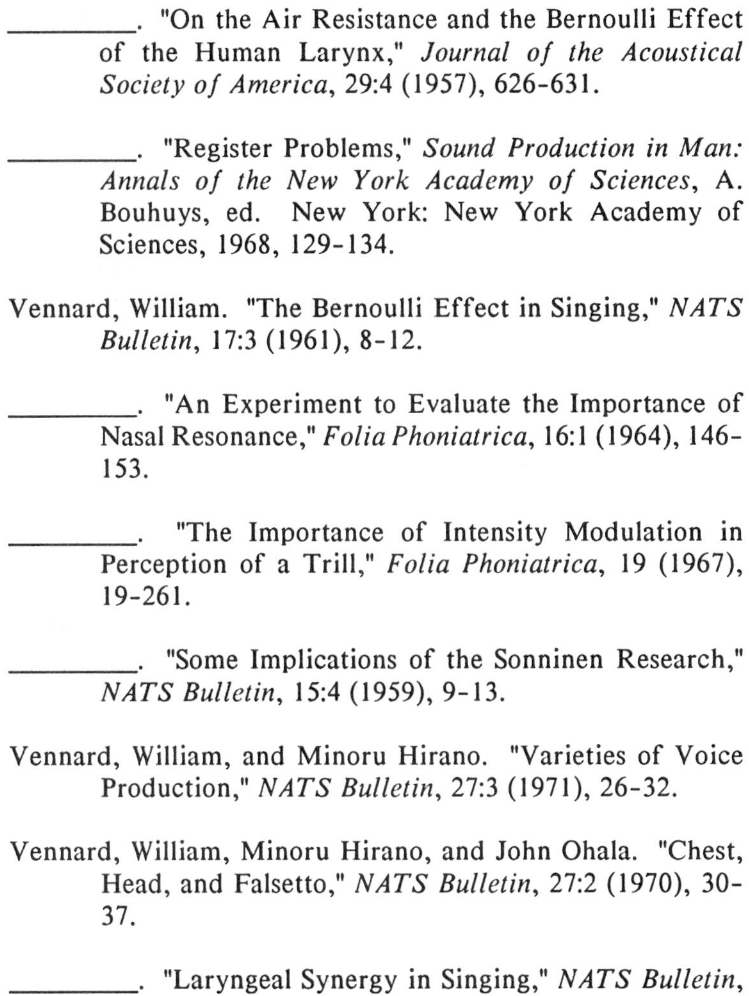

________. "On the Air Resistance and the Bernoulli Effect of the Human Larynx," *Journal of the Acoustical Society of America*, 29:4 (1957), 626-631.

________. "Register Problems," *Sound Production in Man: Annals of the New York Academy of Sciences*, A. Bouhuys, ed. New York: New York Academy of Sciences, 1968, 129-134.

Vennard, William. "The Bernoulli Effect in Singing," *NATS Bulletin*, 17:3 (1961), 8-12.

________. "An Experiment to Evaluate the Importance of Nasal Resonance," *Folia Phoniatrica*, 16:1 (1964), 146-153.

________. "The Importance of Intensity Modulation in Perception of a Trill," *Folia Phoniatrica*, 19 (1967), 19-261.

________. "Some Implications of the Sonninen Research," *NATS Bulletin*, 15:4 (1959), 9-13.

Vennard, William, and Minoru Hirano. "Varieties of Voice Production," *NATS Bulletin*, 27:3 (1971), 26-32.

Vennard, William, Minoru Hirano, and John Ohala. "Chest, Head, and Falsetto," *NATS Bulletin*, 27:2 (1970), 30-37.

________. "Laryngeal Synergy in Singing," *NATS Bulletin*, 27:1 (1970), 16-21.

Vennard, William, and James W. Irwin. "Speech and Song Compared in Sonograms," *NATS Bulletin*, 23:2 (1966), 18-23.

Vennard, William, and Nobuhiko Isshiki. "Coup de Glotte, a Misunderstood Expression," *NATS Bulletin*, 20:3 (1964), 15-18.

Vennard, William, Minoru Hirano, and Bjorn Fritzell. "The Extrinsic Laryngeal Muscles," *NATS Bulletin*, 27:4 (1971), 22-30.

Verdolini-Marston, Katherine, Ingo R. Titze, and David G. Druker. "Changes in Phonation Threshold Pressure with Induced Conditions of Hydration," *Journal of Voice*, 4:2 (1990), 142-151.

Vilkman, Erkki. "An Apparatus for Studying the Role of the Cricothyroid Articulation in the Voice Production of Excised Human Larynges," *Folia Phoniatrica*, 39:4 (1987), 169-177.

Von Leden, Hans. "Objective Measures of Laryngeal Function and Phonation," *Sound Production in Man: Annals of the New York Academy of Sciences*, A. Bouhuys, ed. New York: New York Academy of Sciences, 1968, 56-67.

Waengler, Hans-Heinrich. "Some Remarks and Observations on the Function of the Soft Palate," *NATS Bulletin*, 25:1 (1968), 24-25.

Walker, J. Steven. "An Investigation of the Whistle Register in the Female Voice," *Journal of Voice*, 2:2 (1988), 140-150.

Wang, S. "Sianger's High Formant Associated with Different Larynx Positions in Styles of Singing," *Journal of the Acoustical Society of Japan (E)*, 7:6 (1986), 303-314.

Watson, Peter J., and Thomas J. Hixon. "Respiratory Kinematics in Classical (Opera) Singing," *Journal of Speech and Hearing Research*, 28:1 (1985), 104-122.

Watson, Peter J., Jeannette D. Hoit, Robert W. Lansing, and Thomas J. Hixon. "Abdominal Muscle Activity During Classical Singing," *Journal of Voice*, 3:1 (1989), 36-43.

Watterson, Thomas, Heidi J. Hansen-Magorian, and Stephen C. McFarlane, "A Demographic Description of Laryngeal Contact Ulcer Patients," *Journal of Voice*, 4:1 (1990), 71-75.

Welch, G. F., D. C. Sergeant, and F. MacCurtain. "Xeroradiographic-Electrolaryngographic Analysis of Male Vocal Registers," *Journal of Voice*, 3:3 (1989), 244-256.

Wendahl, R. W., G. P. Moore, and Harry Hollien. "Comments on Vocal Fry," *Folia Phoniatrica*, 15:1 (1963), 251-255.

Whitlock, Weldon. "The Problem of the Passaggio," *NATS Bulletin*, 24:3 (1968), 10-13.

Wilder, Carol. "Vocal Aging," *Care of the Professional Voice*, Transcripts of the Seventh Symposium, Part II, Van Lawrence, ed. New York: Voice Foundation, 1978, 51-59.

Wilder, Carol N., Stephen C. McFarlane, Alfred S. Lavorato, Craig Timberlake, Bonnie Raphael, and Robert T. Sataloff [Panel]. "Voice: Loudness and Projection--Applied Concerns," *Care of the Professional Voice*, Transcripts of the Thirteenth Symposium, Part I, Van Lawrence, ed. New York: Voice Foundation, 1984, 269-278.

Wilson, D. Kenneth. "Vowel Color and Voice Quality," *NATS Bulletin*, 15:1 (1958), 4-7.

Wilson, James E. "Variations of the Laryngo-pharynx in Singing," *NATS Bulletin*, 33:2 (1977), 22-24, 31.

Winckel, Fritz. "How to Measure the Effectiveness of Stage Singers' Voices," *Folia Phoniatrica*, 23:4 (1971), 228-233.

__________. "Measurements of the Acoustic Effectiveness and Quality of Trained Singers' Voices," *NATS Bulletin*, 33:1 (1976), 44.

Wolverton, Vance D. "Classifying Adolescent Singing Voices," *Journal of Research in Singing*, 11:2 (1988), 49-53.

Wooldridge, Warren B. "Is there Nasal Resonance?" *NATS Bulletin*, 13:1 (1956), 28-29.

Yanagihara, Naoku, Yasuo Koike, and Hans von Leden. "Phonation and Respiration," *Folia Phoniatrica*, 18:2 (1966), 323-340.

Yanagisawa, Eiji, Jo Estill, Steven T. Kmucha, and Steven B. Leder. "The Contribution of Ary-Epiglottic Constriction to 'Ringing' Voice Quality--a Videolaryngoscopic Study with Acoustic Analysis," *Journal of Voice*, 3:4 (1989), 342-350.

Zemlin, Willard R. "Notes on the Morphology of the Human Larynx: A Tutorial Exposition," *NATS Bulletin*, 41:1 (1984), 4-10.

Zemlin, Willard R., Robert M. Mason, and Lisa Holstead. "Notes on the Mechanics of Vocal Vibrato," *NATS Bulletin*, 28:2 (1972), 22-26.

Zemlin, Willard R., Patricia Davis, and Cathy Gaza. "Fine Morphology of the Posterior Cricoarytenoid Muscle," *Folia Phoniatrica*, 35:5 (1984), 233-240.

Zender, Wolfgang. "Questions Regarding the Function of External Laryngeal Muscles," *Research Potentials in Voice Physiology*, D. Brewer, ed. Syracuse, NY: State University of New York, 1964, 20-40.

Zwitman, Daniel, and Paul H. Ward. "Variations in Velopharyngeal Closure Assessed by Endoscopy," *Journal of Speech and Hearing Disorders*, 39 (1974), 366-372.

NAME INDEX

SUBJECT INDEX

ABOUT THE AUTHOR

BARBARA M. DOSCHER (D.M.A.) is Professor Emerita of Music at the University of Colorado-Boulder, where she has served as chairwoman of the voice faculty, and presently is an adjunct professor. Her students are singing professionally throughout Europe and the United States. Competitions they have won include the Pavarotti Competition, the Metropolitan Opera National Auditions, and the Mozart Concours International de Chant, and many have been awarded apprenticeships in Chicago, Santa Fe, Houston, Central City, Cincinnati, Tulsa, and Des Moines. She is in high demand as a clinician and has been featured at several national conventions of the National Association of Teachers of Singing. In 1991 and 1992 she was a master teacher at the first two Internship Programs sponsored by the NATS Foundation.

Dr. Doscher has also garnered recognition through her writings. The first edition of *The Functional Unity of the Singing Voice* (Scarecrow, 1988) is in wide use in vocal pedagogy classes throughout the United States and Canada, and her articles have appeared in *The NATS Journal*, *The Choral Journal*, *American Music Teacher*, *Journal of Research in Singing*, and *The Quarterly*.